WEIGHT WA *FREESTYLE COOKBOOK*

2018

The All New Weight Watchers Freestyle Program With 30 days meal plan And A Free Weight Watchers Shopping List for Proven Weight Loss.

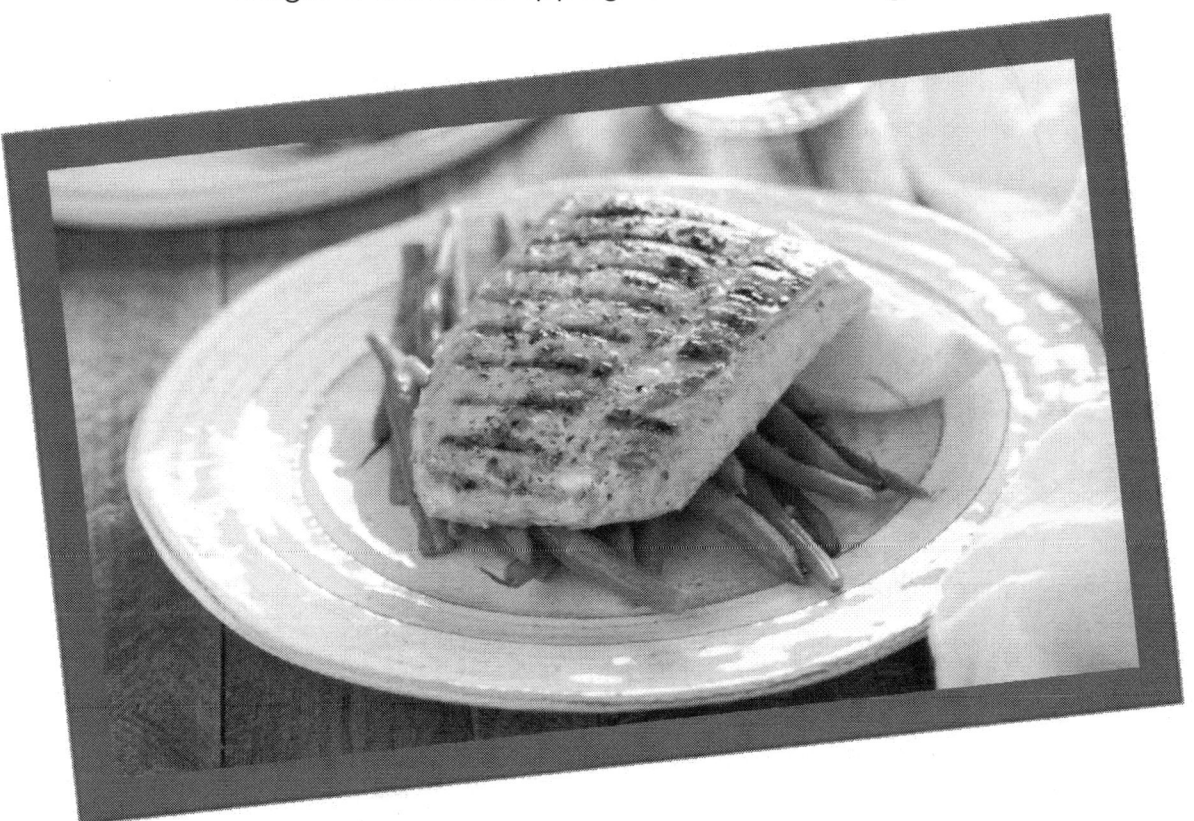

By Michael M

© Copyright 2018 by Michael Smith All rights reserved.
The following eBook is reproduced below with the goal of providing information that is as accurate and as reliable as possible. Regardless, purchasing this eBook can be seen as consent to the fact that both the publisher and the author of this book are in no way experts on the topics discussed within, and that any recommendations or suggestions made herein are for entertainment purposes only. Professionals should be consulted as needed before undertaking any of the action endorsed herein.

This declaration is deemed fair and valid by both the American Bar Association and the Committee of Publishers Association and is legally binding throughout the United States.

Furthermore, the transmission, duplication or reproduction of any of the following work, including precise information, will be considered an illegal act, irrespective whether it is done electronically or in print. The legality extends to creating a secondary or tertiary copy of the work or a recorded copy and is only allowed with express written consent of the Publisher. All additional rights are reserved.

The information in the following pages is broadly considered a truthful and accurate account of facts, and as such, any inattention, use or misuse of the information in question by the reader will render any resulting actions solely under their purview. There are no scenarios in which the publisher or the original author of this work can be in any fashion deemed liable for any hardship or damages that may befall them after undertaking information described herein.

Additionally, the information found on the following pages is intended for informational purposes only and should thus be considered, universal. As befitting its nature, the information presented is without assurance regarding its continued validity or interim quality.

Trademarks that mentioned are done without written consent and can in no way be considered an endorsement from the trademark holder.

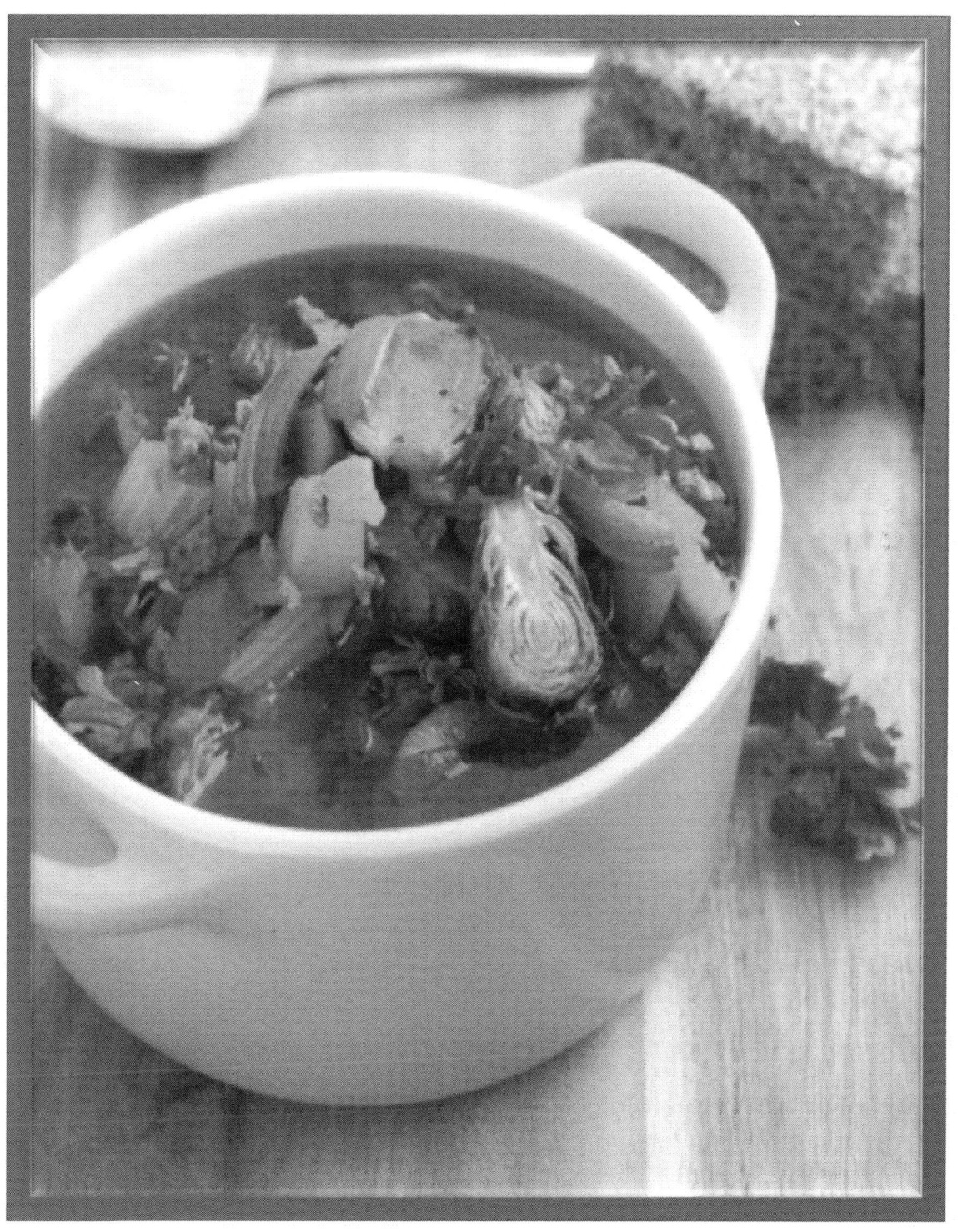

Table of Contents

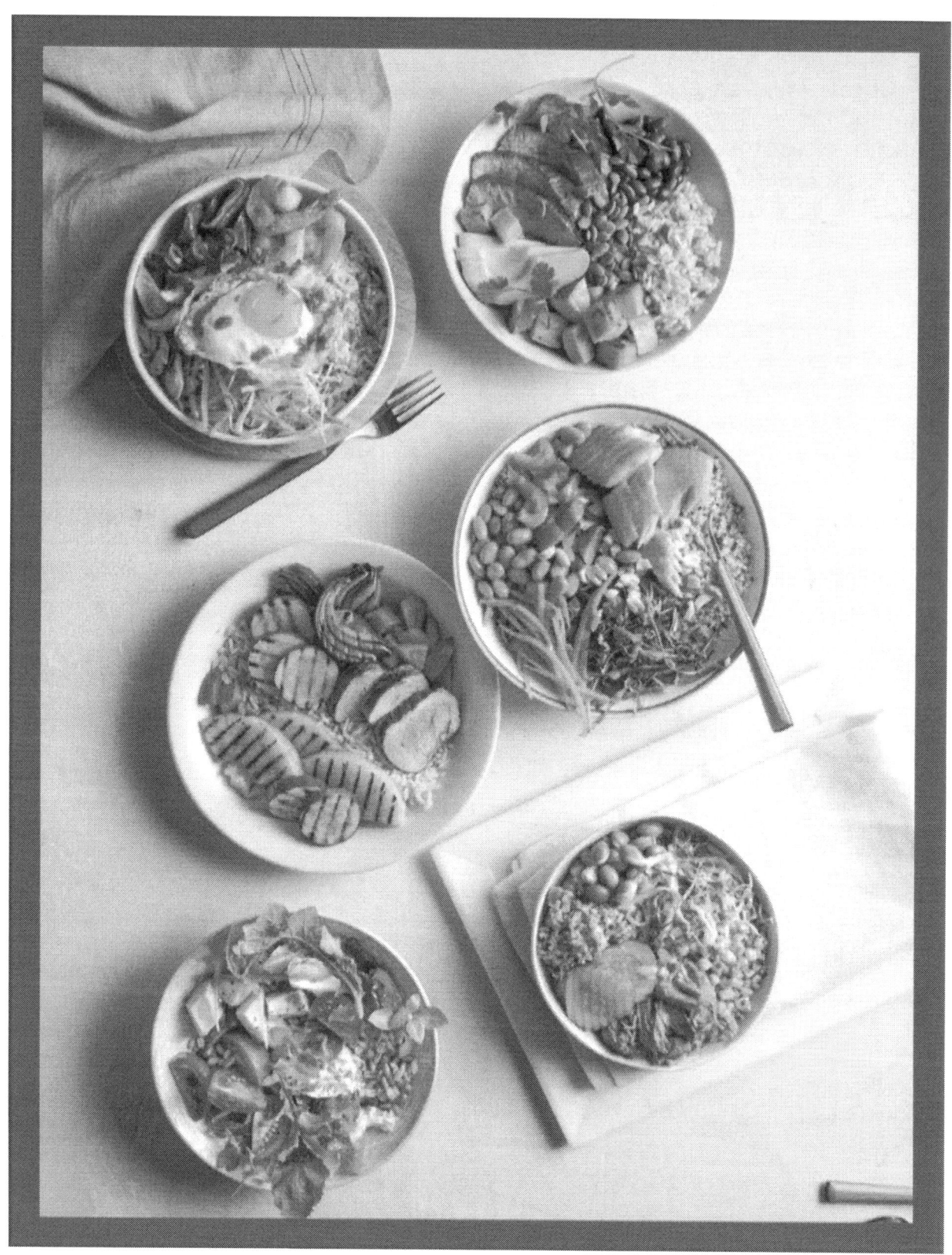

Introduction

The reasons why people lose weight vary from person to person. Over the past two decades, obesity has greatly increased in the USA with statistics showing that more than a third of adults in the USA are overweight. When one is overweight, he or she has a lot of physiological as well as emotional issues, hence people having varied reasons for wanting to lose weight:

- **Being Healthy**

During a research carried out in 2007, half of the target population said their major reason for losing weight was to improve their health. When obese, one is at a risk of developing heart disease, stroke as well as cancer.

- **Mood**

Why is this so? When one is overweight, he or she has insecurities that lead to depression as well as low self-esteem. Moreover, there is also some evidence that disorders related to one's mood and obesity is connected. Also, depression and bipolar disorder may be a precursor to obesity. Past studies have also proved that losing weight leads to improved mood.

- **Fitness**

This is true especially for men who are regarded as being overweight.

- **Wanting to have children**

This is because being overweight can lead to infertility and other complications during pregnancy. As we delve further into weight loss, the amount of weight you need to shed isn't really an important thing as such. You really need to know your real reasons for wanting to lose weight. We may have several reasons for wanting to shed weight, but we may not really realize what they are. When people are asked why they need to lose weight, most of them say: they want to be fit and healthy, they want to be confident, respected, love and so forth.

Consequently, you may start feeling trapped by your weight. You will start being obsessed about what you eat and the amount of exercise you do. There may be people who are leaner than you, but they are less confident, feel less loved and respected. Please be careful to lose weight for the correct reasons. If you have some solid reason for losing weight, you will definitely stick to your diet plan. There are good reasons as well as bad reasons for losing weight. The bad reasons may make you lose weight, but they will not be good enough for a long-term change in one's habits and lifestyle.

Good reasons for losing weight revolve around you while the negative ones revolve around pleasing other people such as:

- Shedding weight so as to attract someone

This may be a great trigger for weight loss; looking nice for someone you would want to be with. However, ask yourself what happens if this person does not exist in your life anymore? You will definitely lose your motivation for losing weight.

- Weight loss to boost health

This will be about you and it does not depend on what someone else thinks, says or does.

- Being referred to as overweight

Insults could motivate you to change your appearance. However, you don't need to change so as to impress someone.

In short, losing weight needs to be about you and nobody else. This is the only way to maintain your motivation and be focused on your goals.

Many people, including you, who is reading this, don't understand the main reasons why they want to lose weight. Your reasons for weight loss should be deeper and meaningful; they need to originate from your inner self. As soon as you have your valid reasons for losing weight, jot them down on an index card. Place them by your bedside and read them when you wake up and before retiring to bed.

Furthermore, you can also keep a copy at work and another in your wallet as a constant reminder of your goals.

You should also know that weight-loss goals, determine the difference between success and failure. Goals that are well-planned will keep you focused and motivated. Goals that are not realistic and overly ambitious will definitely undermine your efforts. Below are tips on losing weight:

- Concentrate on process goals

An outcome goal could be what you hope to achieve in the end. Even though this goal may give you a target, it does not guide you on how to achieve it. A process goal is a vital step in achieving whatever you desire. For instance, a process goal could be eating five portions of fruits or veggies on a daily basis, walking for half an hour daily or maybe drinking water after every meal. Process goals are particularly helpful when losing weight because you will focus on changing behaviors and habits that are important in weight loss.

- Set smart goals
1. They need to be specific- a good goal needs to have specific details.
2. They need to be measurable- if you can measure a goal, then you can objectively determine how successful you are at achieving the goal.
3. They need to be achievable- For instance, if your schedule doesn't allow you to spend an hour at the gym, then this is an unattainable goal.
4. They need to be realistic
- Your goals also need to be track-able
- Have long-term and short-term goals
- Don't try to be perfect

Setbacks are a natural part of behavior change. No one who is successful has never experienced setbacks. Identify potential barriers.

- Reassess and adjust goals as required

Weight Watchers

People used to strive for ways to find food. As the world advanced, we have so much of food that we don't know how to stop consuming it. That's where diet programs come in. The market is now congested with different dietary programs, all making claims of being the best. But few have achieved the heights that Weight Watchers has. And to know the secret behind Weight Watchers success we take an in-depth look into what makes it stand out.

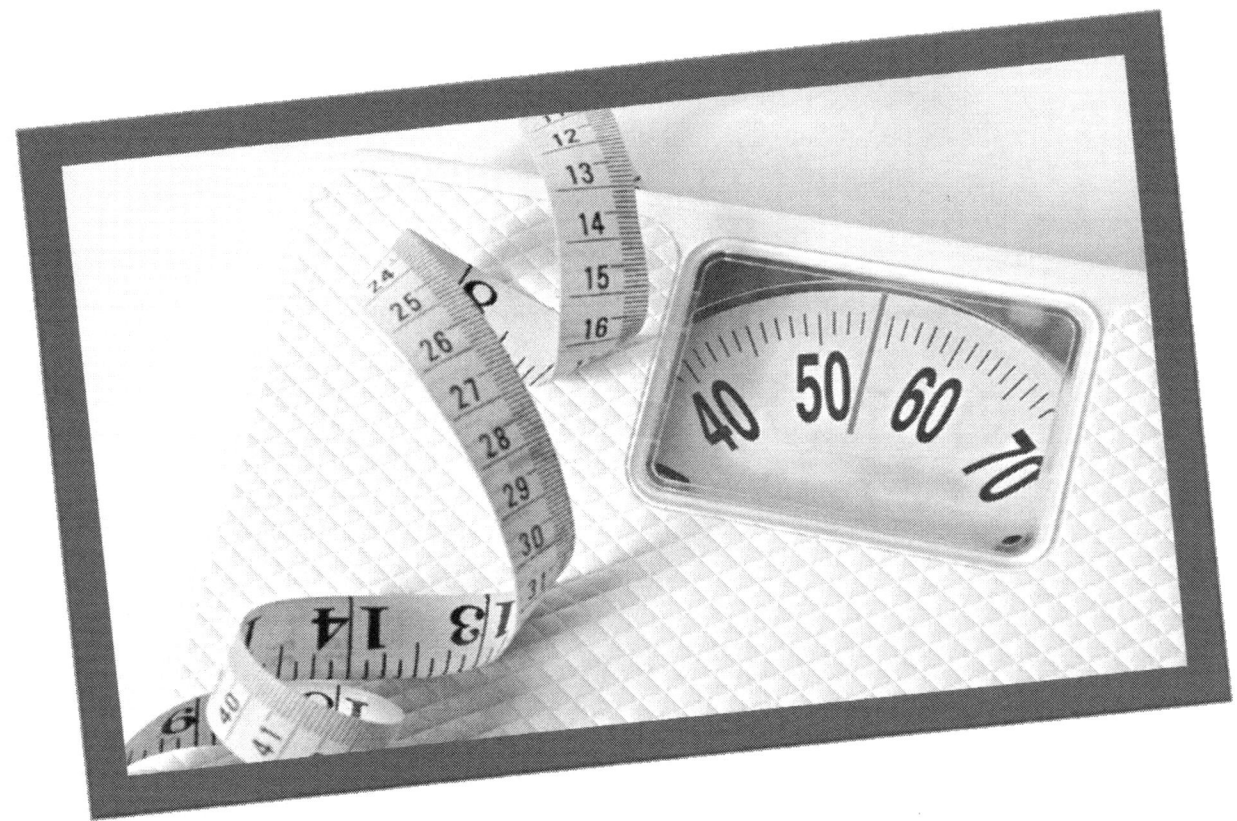

Weight Watchers FreeStyle 2018

Based on the successful SmartPoints® system, WW Freestyle offers more than 200 zero Points® foods—including eggs, skinless chicken breast, fish and seafood, corn, beans, peas, and so much more—to multiply your meal and menu possibilities. And it makes life simpler, too: You can forget about weighing, measuring, or tracking those zero Points foods.

All New Freestyle Recipes

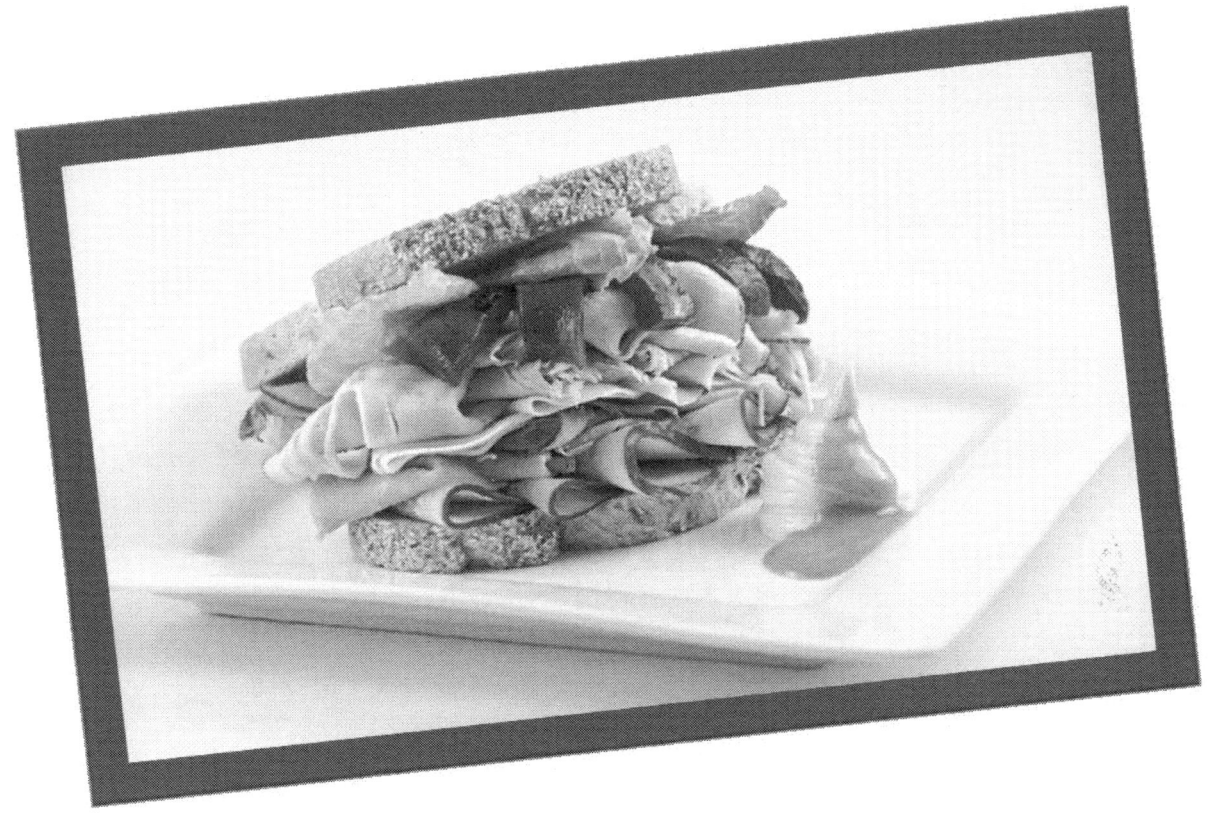

OFS - Crock Pot Chicken Cacciatore

(Prep time:10 min | Cook time:10 min | Total time:20 min | Serves: 5)

INGREDIENTS:

- 8 bone-in, skinless chicken thighs (about 5-ounces each), fat trimmed- in the photos for this recipe, you'll notice that I actually used 5 full chicken legs (drumstick and thigh) instead
- 3/4 teaspoon kosher salt
- freshly ground black pepper
- cooking spray
- 5 garlic cloves, finely chopped
- 1/2 large onion, chopped
- 1 28-ounce can crushed tomatoes
- 1/2 medium red bell pepper, chopped
- 1/2 medium green bell pepper, chopped
- 4 ounce sliced shiitake mushrooms

- 1 sprig of fresh thyme
- 1 sprig of fresh oregano
- 1 bay leaf
- 1 tablespoon chopped fresh parsley (I omitted this)
- freshly grated Parmesan cheese, for serving (optional)

DIRECTIONS:

1. Season the chicken with salt and pepper to taste. Heat a large nonstick skillet over medium-high heat. Coat with cooking spray, add the chicken, and cook until browned- 2 to 3 minutes per side. Transfer to your slow cooker.
2. Reduce the heat under the skillet to medium and coat with more cooking spray. Add the garlic and onion and cook, stirring, until soft- 3 to 4 minutes.
3. Transfer to the slow cooker and add the tomatoes, bell peppers, mushrooms, thyme, oregano and bay leaf. Stir to combine.
4. Cover and cook on high for 4 hours or on low for 8 hours.
5. Discard the bay leaf and transfer the chicken to a large plate. Pull the chicken meat from the bones (discard the bones), shred the meat, and return it to the sauce.
6. Stir in the parsley (if using). If desired, serve topped with Parmesan cheese.

Nutritional information per serving: Calories: 220, Fat: 6g, Sat Fat: 1.5g, Cholesterol: 123mg, Sodium: 319mg, Carbohydrates: 10g, Fiber: 2g, Sugar: 6g, Protein: 31g

0 SmartPoints on FreeStyle Plan or FlexPlan

OFS - Succotash Bean Soup

(Prep time:10 min | Cook time:10 min | Total time:20 min | Serves: 5)
(12 approximately 1 cup servings)
Ingredients:
2 cans white beans (rinsed and drained)
2 cans Lima beans (rinsed and drained)
2 cans corn kernels drained
1 carton low sodium vegetable broth
12 slices Canadian bacon chopped into small pieces
Season to taste
Instructions

Dump all ingredients into a large crockpot. Stir gently to evenly mix ingredients. Cook on low 6-8 hours. This is zero points...you have enough left for cornbread!

0 SmartPoints on FreeStyle Plan or FlexPlan

0FS - Crock Pot Chicken Taco Chili

(Prep time:10 min | Cook time:10 min | Total time:6 h | Serves: 5)

INGREDIENTS:

- 1 small onion, chopped
- 1 (15.5 oz.) can black beans, drained
- 1 (15.5 oz.) can kidney beans, drained
- 1 (8 oz.) can tomato sauce
- 10 oz. package frozen corn kernels
- 2 (10 oz.) cans diced tomatoes w/chilies
- 4 oz. can chopped green chili peppers, chopped
- 1 packet reduced sodium taco seasoning or homemade (see below)
- 1 tbsp. cumin
- 1 tbsp. chili powder
- 24 oz. (3) boneless skinless chicken breasts
- 1/4 cup chopped fresh cilantro

To make your own taco seasoning, omit the packet, cumin and chili powder above and use below instead:

- 1 1/2 tablespoons cumin
- 1 1/2 tablespoons chili powder
- 1/4 teaspoon garlic powder
- 1/4 teaspoon onion powder
- 1/4 teaspoon dried oregano
- 1/2 teaspoon paprika
- 1 teaspoon kosher salt
- 1/2 teaspoon black pepper

DIRECTIONS:

1. Combine beans, onion, chili peppers, corn, tomato sauce, diced tomato, cumin, chili powder and taco seasoning in a slow cooker and mix well.
2. Nestle the chicken in to completely cover and cook on LOW for 8 to 10 hours or on HIGH for 4 to 6 hours.

3. Half hour before serving, remove chicken and shred.
4. Return chicken to slow cooker and stir in.
5. Top with fresh cilantro and your favorite toppings!

NUTRITION INFORMATION

Yield: 10 servings, Serving Size: About 1 cup
- **Amount Per Serving:**

Calories: 220, Total Fat: 3g, Saturated Fat: g
Carbohydrates: 28g, Fiber: 8.5g, Sugar: 6g, Protein: 21g

0 SmartPoints on FreeStyle Plan

OFS - Authentic Shoyu Ahi Poke

(Prep time:5 min | Cook time:0 min | Total time:5 min | Serves: 5)
TOTAL TIME: 5 minutes

Shoyu Ahi Poke is the traditional Hawaiian dish of raw fish seasoned with soy sauce and sesame oil.

INGREDIENTS:
- 1 lbs. sushi grade tuna, cut into 3/4 inch cubes
- 1/4 cup thin sliced onions
- 1/2 cup sliced scallions, green parts only
- 2 tbsp. reduced sodium soy sauce* (use coconut aminos for Whole30/Paleo)
- 1 teaspoon sesame oil
- 1/2 teaspoon sambal oelek or sriracha

DIRECTIONS:
1. In a medium bowl combine all the ingredients and gently fold until mixed well.
2. Serve immediately or cover tight and refrigerate for up to a day.
3. If you let it marinate, you may need to add another splash of soy sauce to taste.

*use gluten-free soy sauce for gluten-free diets.

NUTRITION INFORMATION

Yield: 4 servings, Serving Size: 1/4 lbs. poke only (veggies extra)
- **Amount Per Serving:**

Calories: 166, Total Fat: 4g, Saturated Fat: g, Carbohydrates: 2.5g
Fiber: 0.5g, Sugar: 0.6g, Protein: 28.5g

0 SmartPoints on FreeStyle Plan

OFS - Red Pepper Muffin Tin Eggs

(Prep time:10 min | Cook time:40 min | Total time:50 min | Serves: 12)
Ingredients

- 12 eggs
- 1 teaspoon Montreal Steak Seasoning Blend
- 1 red, orange, or green pepper, diced
- ½ pound 99% fat-free ground turkey breast
- ½ teaspoon sage
- ½ teaspoon salt
- ½ teaspoon black pepper
- ¼ teaspoon red pepper flakes
- ¼ teaspoon marjoram
- Non-Stick Cooking Spray

Instructions

1. Preheat oven to 350 degrees.
2. Spray a muffin tin with non-stick spray.
3. Spray a large non-stick skillet with non-stick spray. On medium heat cook ground turkey, sage, salt, black pepper, red pepper flakes, and marjoram for 7-10 minutes or until cooked through. Stir consistently to prevent sticking.
4. While turkey is cooking, in a large bowl, beat eggs and Montreal steak seasoning together until well mixed and fluffy (2-3 minutes). Stir in diced bell pepper.
5. Once the turkey is cooked through, spoon into the muffin tins spreading equally between each muffin tin.
6. Pour egg mixture over the turkey filling ¾ of the way full.
7. Bake at 350 degrees for 30 minutes.

Makes 6 Servings (2 muffin tin eggs per serving)
0 SmartPoints on FreeStyle Plan

OFS - Slow Cooked Chicken Verde

INGREDIENTS

1 Pound Boneless Skinless Chicken Breasts
6 Tomatillos peeled and quartered
2 Jalapenos Seeded
1/2 White Onion quartered
2 Tablespoons Minced Garlic
1/2 Cup Fat-Free Low Sodium Chicken Broth
1 Tablespoon Cumin
1 Teaspoon Salt
1 Teaspoon Black Pepper

DIRECTIONS

In blender purée all ingredients except for chicken until a slightly chunky.

- Place chicken in bottom of crock pot and pour purée over top
- Cook on low heat for 6 hours
- Shred chicken and serve with extra sauce over top

Makes 6 servings
0 SmartPoints on FreeStyle Plan

0FS - Beef Veggie Lentil Soup

(Prep time:10 min | Cook time:10 min | Total time:20 min | Serves: 5)

INGREDIENTS:

- 10 cups reduced-sodium beef broth

- 1 pound dried lentils, picked over, rinsed & drained

- 4 large carrots, peeled and finely chopped

- 1 large onion, peeled and finely chopped

- 2 large celery stalks, finely chopped

- 2 bay leaves

- One 14.5-ounce can diced tomatoes, with juice

- 1 tablespoon red wine vinegar

- freshly ground black pepper

- 1 to 2 cups hot water

- chopped chives for garnish, optional

DIRECTIONS:

1. In a large pot, combine the broth, lentils, carrots, onions, celery, and bay leaves; bring to a boil.Reduce the heat, and simmer, covered, stirring occasionally, until the lentils and vegetables are tender (about 30 minutes).

2. Add the tomatoes (with juice), vinegar and pepper.Add the water (amount depending on how much soupy broth you desire).Cover and cook, stirring occasionally, until the flavors have blended, 10 minutes.

3. Sprinkle individual servings with chives, if desired.

Nutritional Information per Serving (serving size 1 3/4 cups) Calories: 261, Fat: 2g, Saturated Fat: 0, Cholesterol: 0, Sodium: 364mg, Carbohydrates: 44g, Fiber 15g, Protein: 19g, Calcium: 72mg

0 SmartPoints on FreeStyle Plan or FlexPlan

OFS - Succotash Bean Soup

(Prep time:10 min | Cook time:10 min | Total time:20 min | Serves: 5)

(12 approximately 1 cup servings)

Ingredients:

2 cans white beans (rinsed and drained)
2 cans Lima beans (rinsed and drained)
2 cans corn kernels drained
1 carton low sodium vegetable broth
12 slices Canadian bacon chopped into small pieces
Season to taste

Instructions

Dump all ingredients into a large crockpot. Stir gently to evenly mix ingredients. Cook on low 6-8 hours. This is zero points...you have enough left for cornbread!

0 SmartPoints on FreeStyle Plan or FlexPlan

OFS - Slow Cooker Black Beans

(Prep time:5 min | Cook time:8 h | Total time:8 h 5 min | Serves: 10)
Ingredients
- 2 cups dry black beans
- 1 onion, quartered
- 4 garlic cloves, peeled
- 2 jalapeno peppers, whole
- 1 bay leaf
- 1 tsp. salt

Nutritional Facts
Serving Size:
1/2 cup
Amount Per Serving
Calories 140, Total Fat 1g, Saturated Fat 0g, Total Carbohydrate 26g
Dietary Fiber 6g, Sugars 1g, Protein 9g
Directions
1. Add everything to the slow cooker. Cover the beans with water or stock until there is one inch of water over the beans.
2. Cook on low for 8 hours.

0 SmartPoints on FreeStyle Plan or FlexPlan

OFS - Crockpot Tomato Balsamic Chicken

(Prep time:10 min | Cook time:4 h | Total time:4 h, 10 min | Serves: 6)
Ingredients
- 2 lbs. boneless and skinless chicken breast
- 28 oz. canned diced tomatoes, half of liquid drained
- 1 sweet onion, sliced thin
- 4 garlic cloves, minced
- 3 tbsp. balsamic vinegar (plus more for serving)
- 1 tbsp. Italian seasoning
- 6 cups fresh spinach
- Salt and pepper

Nutritional Facts
Serving Size:
3/4 cup
Amount Per Serving

Calories 227

Calories from Fat 14

Total Fat 2g

Saturated Fat 0g

Total Carbohydrate 12g

Dietary Fiber 3g

Sugars 7g

Protein 35g

Directions

1. Add the chicken to the slow cooker. Season with salt and pepper. Stir in the remaining ingredients except the spinach.
2. Cook on low for 4 hours adding the spinach during the last 30 minutes of cooking.

0 SmartPoints on FreeStyle Plan or FlexPlan

0FS - Zero Points Bean Soup:

0 WW Freestyle Smart Points (12 approximately 1 cup servings)

Ingredients:

- 2 cans white beans (rinsed and drained)
- 2 cans Lima beans (rinsed and drained)
- 2 cans corn kernels drained
- 1 carton low sodium vegetable broth
- 12 slices Canadian Bacon chopped into small pieces
- Season to taste,

Directions:

1. Dump all ingredients into a large crockpot.
2. Stir gently to evenly mix ingredients.
3. Cook on low 6-8 hours. This is zero points...you have enough left for cornbread!

0FS - Simple Garden Vegetable Soup

(Prep time:15 min | Cook time:30 min | Total time:45 min | Serves: 5)

Ingredients

- 1/2 cup chopped onion

- 1/2 cup chopped carrots

- 1/2 cup chopped celery

- 2 garlic cloves, pressed

- 4 cups fat-free broth of your choice

- 1 can (14-1/2 ounces) diced tomatoes

- 1 cup chopped cabbage

- 1 cup chopped spinach or kale

- 1 tablespoon tomato paste

- 1/2 teaspoon dried basil (or more to taste)

- 1/2 teaspoon dried thyme (or more to taste)

- 1/2 teaspoon salt

- 1 cup chopped zucchini

- Chopped parsley or basil for garnish (optional)

Instructions

1. Spray a large saucepan or soup pot with nonstick cooking spray. Add the onion, carrot and celery and cook over low heat, stirring often until the vegetables have softened.

2. Add the garlic and stir for another minute.

3. Add the broth, tomatoes, cabbage, spinach, tomato paste, basil, thyme and salt and bring to a boil over medium high heat. Lower the heat, cover the pot and simmer gently for about 15 minutes.

4. Add the zucchini and cook until softened, 3 - 5 minutes more.

5. Stir in chopped fresh parsley or basil just before serving if desired.

Slow Cooker Instructions

1. Place everything in your slow cooker, cover and cook on LOW until tender, 6 to 8 hours.

Nutrition Facts
Amount per Serving (1 cup)
Calories 41Calories from Fat 8

(0 PointsPlus | 0 SmartPoints | 0 SmartPoints on FreeStyle Plan or FlexPlan)

OFS - Slow Cooker Shredded Chicken

(Prep time:5 min | Cook time:4 h | Total time:6h 5 min | Serves: 3)

Ingredients

- 3-4 lbs. chicken breast , raw
- 4-5 cups low sodium chicken broth
- 3-4 tabs dried minced onion
- 1 tabs garlic powder
- 1 1/2 tsp celery salt
- 1 tsp pepper

Instructions

1. In a 6-quart slow cooker, add chicken breasts, broth, and seasonings.
2. Cook on low for 6 hours, or high for 4 hours.
3. Remove and transfer onto a cutting board, let cool, and shred into pieces. (Or shred with mixer)

Recipe Notes

Serving size: 3 oz.

0 SmartPoints on FreeStyle Plan or FlexPlan

OFS - Beef Veggie Lentil Soup

(Prep time:10 min | Cook time:10 min | Total time:20 min | Serves: 5)

INGREDIENTS:

- 10 cups reduced-sodium beef broth
- 1 pound dried lentils, picked over, rinsed & drained
- 4 large carrots, peeled and finely chopped
- 1 large onion, peeled and finely chopped
- 2 large celery stalks, finely chopped
- 2 bay leaves
- One 14.5-ounce can diced tomatoes, with juice
- 1 tablespoon red wine vinegar
- freshly ground black pepper
- 1 to 2 cups hot water
- chopped chives for garnish, optional

DIRECTIONS:

4. In a large pot, combine the broth, lentils, carrots, onions, celery, and bay leaves; bring to a boil.Reduce the heat, and simmer, covered, stirring occasionally, until the lentils and vegetables are tender (about 30 minutes).
5. Add the tomatoes (with juice), vinegar and pepper.Add the water (amount depending on how much soupy broth you desire).Cover and cook, stirring occasionally, until the flavors have blended, 10 minutes.
6. Sprinkle individual servings with chives, if desired.

Nutritional Information per Serving (serving size 1 3/4 cups) Calories: 261, Fat: 2g, Saturated Fat: 0, Cholesterol: 0, Sodium: 364mg, Carbohydrates: 44g, Fiber 15g, Protein: 19g, Calcium: 72mg
0 SmartPoints on FreeStyle Plan

0FS - Grilled Lime Shrimp Kebabs

(Prep time:10 min | Cook time:20 min | Total time:30 min | Serves: 4)
INGREDIENTS:
- 32 jumbo raw shrimp, peeled and deveined (17.5 oz. after peeled)
- 3 cloves garlic, crushed
- 24 slices (about 3) large limes, very thinly sliced into rounds (optional)
- olive oil cooking spray (I use my mister)
- 1 tsp kosher salt
- 1 1/2 tsp ground cumin
- 1/4 cup chopped fresh cilantro, divided
- 16 bamboo skewers soaked in water 1 hour
- 1 lime cut into 8 wedges

DIRECTIONS:
1. Heat the grill on medium heat and spray the grates with oil.
2. Season the shrimp with garlic, cumin, salt and half of the cilantro in a medium bowl.
3. Beginning and ending with shrimp, thread the shrimp and folded lime slices onto 8 pairs of parallel skewers to make 8 kebabs total.
4. Grill the shrimp, turning occasionally, until shrimp is opaque throughout, about 1 to 2 minutes on each side.

5. Top with remaining cilantro and fresh squeezed lime juice before serving.

NUTRITION INFORMATION

Yield: 8 servings, Serving Size: 1 kebab
- **Amount Per Serving:**

Calories: 74, Total Fat: 1g, Saturated Fat: g

Carbohydrates: 3g, Fiber: 1g, Sugar: 0g, Protein: 13g

0 SmartPoints on FreeStyle Plan

0FS - Turkey Veggie Soup

(Prep time:20 min | Cook time:20 min | Total time:40 min | Serves: 6)

INGREDIENTS:
- 1 cup finely chopped celery (about 2 stalks)
- 1/2 cup finely chopped onion
- 1 1/2 teaspoons minced garlic
- 1 1/2 pounds 99% fat-free ground turkey breast
- 3 cups fat free beef or chicken broth
- 1 cup sliced carrot (about 2 large)
- 1/2 cup trimmed fresh green beans, cut in 1-inch lengths
- 1/2 cup frozen whole-kernel corn
- 1 1/2 teaspoons ground cumin
- 1 teaspoon chili powder
- 2 whole bay leaves
- One 15-ounce can kidney beans, rinsed and drained
- One 14.5-ounce can diced tomatoes and green chiles, undrained
- 6 tablespoons shredded Monterey Jack cheese, optional

DIRECTIONS:
1. Heat a Dutch oven over medium-high heat. Coat pan with cooking spray.
2. Add celery, onion, garlic and turkey. Cook 5 minutes or until ground turkey is browned, stirring to crumble. Add 3 cups of beef stock and remaining ingredients except cheese; bring to a boil. Cover, reduce heat, and simmer 20 minutes or until vegetables are tender. Discard bay leaves.
3. Ladle 1 1/2 cups soup into each of 6 bowls; top each serving with 1 Tablespoon of cheese.

Nutritional Information per serving: (Serving size: 1 1/2 cups soup- with 1 tablespoon of cheese) Calories: 265, Fat: 5g, Saturated Fat: 2g, Sugar: 7g, Sodium: 1789mg, Fiber: 7.5g, Protein: 27g, Cholesterol: 55mg, Carbohydrates per serving: 29g
0 SmartPoints on FreeStyle Plan

0FS - Chicken Enchilada Stuffed Zucchini

(Prep time:10 min | Cook time:10 min | Total time:20 min | Serves: 8)
Ingredients:
For the enchilada sauce:
- olive oil spray
- 2 garlic cloves, minced
- 1 or 2 tbsp. chipotle chile in adobo sauce, more if you like it spicy
- 1-1/2 cups tomato sauce
- 1/2 tsp chipotle chili powder
- 1/2 tsp ground cumin
- 2/3 cup fat-free low-sodium chicken broth
- kosher salt and fresh pepper to taste

For the zucchini boats:
- 4 (about 32 oz. total) medium zucchini
- 1 tsp oil
- 1/2 cup green onions, chopped
- 3 cloves garlic, crushed
- 1/2 cup diced green bell pepper
- 1/4 cup chopped cilantro
- 8 oz. cooked shredded chicken breast
- 1 tsp cumin
- 1/2 tsp dried oregano
- 1/2 tsp chipotle chili powder
- 3 tbsp. water or fat free chicken broth
- 1 tbsp. tomato paste
- salt and pepper to taste

For the Topping:
- 3/4 cup reduced fat shredded sharp cheddar
- chopped scallions and cilantro for garnish

Directions:

For the enchilada sauce: In a medium saucepan, **spray** oil and **sauté** garlic. **Add** chipotle chiles, chili powder, cumin, chicken broth, tomato sauce, salt and pepper. Bring to a boil. **Reduce** the heat to low and **simmer** for 5-10 minutes. Set aside until ready to use.

For the Zucchini Boats: Bring a large pot of water to boil.

Preheat oven to 400°. **Cut** zucchini in half lengthwise and using a small spoon or melon baller, **scoop** out flesh, leaving 1/4" thick. **Chop** the scooped out flesh of the zucchini in small pieces and set aside.

Drop the zucchini halves in boiling water and cook 1 minute; **remove** from water.

In a large sauté pan, **heat** oil and **add** onion, garlic and bell pepper. **Cook** on medium-low heat for about 2-3 minutes, until onions are translucent. **Add** chopped zucchini and cilantro; **season** with salt and pepper and **cook** about 4 minutes. **Add** the cumin, oregano, chili powder, water, and tomato paste and cook a few more minutes, then **add** in chicken; **mix** and cook 3 more minutes.

Place 1/4 cup of the enchilada sauce on the bottom of a large (or 2 small) baking dish, and place zucchini halves cut side up. Using a spoon, **fill** each hollowed zucchini with 1/3 cup chicken mixture, pressing firmly.

Top each with 2 tablespoons of enchilada sauce, and 1 1/2 tablespoons each of shredded cheese.

Cover with foil and **bake** 35 minutes until cheese is melted and zucchini is cooked through.

Top with scallions and cilantro for garnish and serve with low fat sour cream if desired.

Servings: 8 • **Size:** 1 zucchini boat • **Calories:** 116 • **Fat:** 3.5 g • **Protein:** 12 g • **Carb:** 11 g • **Fiber:** 3 g • **Sugar:** 4.5 g **Sodium:** 410 mg (without salt)
(3 PointsPlus | 3 SmartPoints | 0 SmartPoints on FreeStyle Plan or FlexPlan)

OFS - Turkey Pumpkin Chili

(Prep time:20 min | Cook time:1 h | Total time:1 h20 min | Serves: 8)
INGREDIENTS:

- 1 pound 99% lean ground turkey
- 3/4 cup chopped onions

- 1/2 cup chopped green bell peppers
- 2 cloves garlic, minced
- 2 (14.5 ounce) cans diced tomatoes, with liquid
- 1 (15 ounce) can unsweetened pure pumpkin puree
- 1 (15 ounce) can kidney beans, with liquid
- 1 (15 ounce) can Great Northern beans, with liquid
- 1 (15 ounce) can tomato sauce
- 1 (4 ounce) can diced green chiles
- 2 teaspoons ground chili powder
- 1 1/2 teaspoons ground cumin (or more to taste)
- 1 teaspoon salt
- 1/2 teaspoon ground black pepper
- 1 1/2 teaspoons oregano
- 1/2 cup water

DIRECTIONS:

1. Brown meat in large pot. Remove meat and place on paper towels to remove excess fat. Wipe any remaining fat from the pot and coat pot with cooking spray.
2. Sauté onion, bell pepper and garlic; sauté until tender. Return meat to pot. Add all remaining ingredients and stir to combine. Simmer 30 minutes to 1 hour. If chili is too thick for you, add more water, and adjust seasonings as needed.

Nutritional Information per serving (Serving size: Recipe divided into 8 equal portions) Calories: 276, Fat: 6g, Saturated Fat: 1.5g, Sugar: 4g, Fiber: 5.25g, Protein: 20g, Carbohydrates: 39g

0 SmartPoints on FreeStyle Plan

0FS – GreekStyle Chickpea Salad

0 WW Freestyle SP per serving.

INGREDIENTS

- 2 (15 ounce) cans chickpea, drained and rinsed
- 1 small tomato, chopped
- ¼ cup finely chopped red onion
- ½ teaspoon sugar
- ¼ cup reduced fat crumbled feta cheese
- ½ tablespoon lemon juice
- ½ tablespoon red wine vinegar

- 1 tablespoon plain nonfat Greek Yogurt
- 2 cloves garlic, minced
- ¼ teaspoon salt
- ¼ teaspoon pepper
- 1-2 tablespoons cilantro

INSTRUCTIONS
1. Drain and rinse the chickpeas and place in a medium bowl.
2. Toss in the rest of the ingredients until chickpeas are evenly coated and all of the ingredients are mixed well.
3. Serve immediately and refrigerate any leftovers.

Nutrition Information
- Serves: 8 servings
- Serving size: ½ cup
- Calories: 192
- Fat: 4 g
- Saturated fat: 1 g
- Carbohydrates: 32 g
- Sugar: 6 g
- Fiber: 8 g
- Protein: 10 g
- Cholesterol: 4 mg

0FS - Mexican Chicken Soup

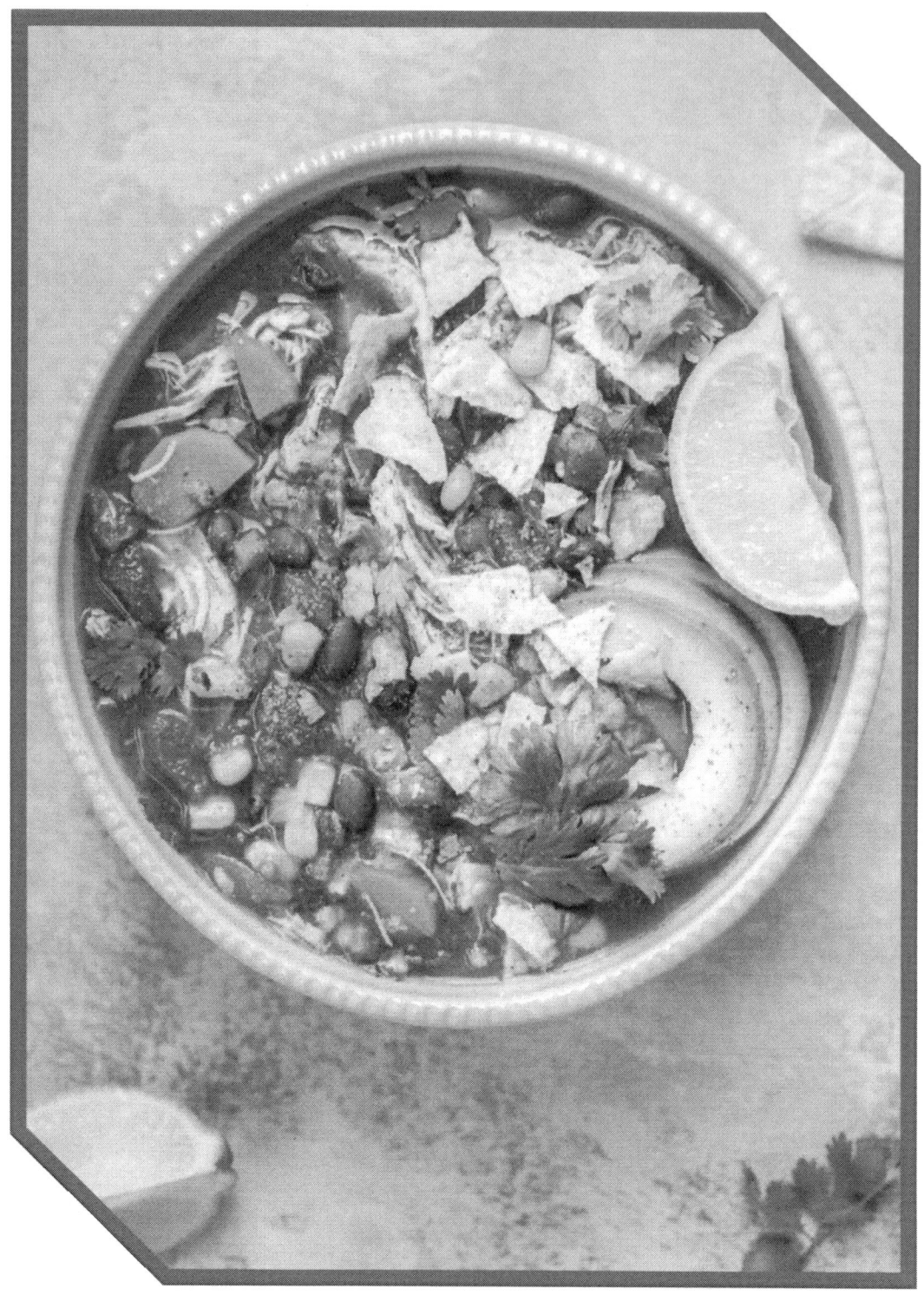

(Prep time:15 min | Cook time:6 H | Total time:6 H 15 min | Serves: 10)
Ingredients

- 2 cups salsa chicken shredded

- 1 small onion chopped

- 2 cloves garlic crushed

- 1 20 ounces can crushed tomatoes

- 1 12 ounces can great northern beans

- 1 12 ounces can red kidney beans

- 1 cup frozen whole kernel corn

- 6 cups fat-free chicken stock

- 1 tablespoon cumin

- 1 teaspoon garlic powder

- 1 teaspoon onion powder

- 1 teaspoon paprika

- 1 teaspoon chili powder

- 1 teaspoon black pepper

- 1 teaspoon salt

Instructions

1. Mix all ingredients together in large Crockpot.

2. Cook on low heat for 6 hours or high heat for 3 hours.

3. Serve alone or with tortilla chips or strips as desired.

0 SmartPoints on FreeStyle Plan or FlexPlan

OFS - Slow Cook Chicken Cacciatore

INGREDIENTS:

- 8 bone-in, skinless chicken thighs
- 3/4 teaspoon kosher salt
- freshly ground black pepper
- cooking spray
- 5 garlic cloves, finely chopped
- 1/2 large onion, chopped
- 1 28-ounce can crushed tomatoes
- 1/2 medium red bell pepper, chopped
- 1/2 medium green bell pepper, chopped
- 4 ounce sliced shiitake mushrooms
- 1 sprig of fresh thyme
- 1 sprig of fresh oregano
- 1 bay leaf
- 1 tablespoon chopped fresh parsley (I omitted this)
- freshly grated Parmesan cheese, for serving (optional)

DIRECTIONS:

1. Season the chicken with salt and pepper to taste. Heat a large nonstick skillet over medium-high heat.
2. Coat with cooking spray, add the chicken, and cook until browned- 2 to 3 minutes per side. Transfer to your slow cooker.
3. Reduce the heat under the skillet to medium and coat with more cooking spray. Add the garlic and onion and cook, stirring, until soft- 3 to 4 minutes.
4. Transfer to the slow cooker and add the tomatoes, bell peppers, mushrooms, thyme, oregano and bay leaf. Stir to combine.
5. Cover and cook on high for 4 hours or on low for 8 hours.
6. Discard the bay leaf and transfer the chicken to a large plate. Pull the chicken meat from the bones (discard the bones), shred the meat, and return it to the sauce.
7. Stir in the parsley (if using). If desired, serve topped with Parmesan cheese.

Nutritional information per serving: Calories: 220, Fat: 6g, Sat Fat: 1.5g, Cholesterol: 123mg, Sodium: 319mg, Carbohydrates: 10g, Fiber: 2g, Sugar: 6g, Protein: 31g

Weight Watchers POINTS: Freestyle SmartPoints: 0 (but only if you use chicken breast instead of thighs)

1FS - Healthy Tuna Salad Wraps

(Prep time:5 min | Cook time:5 min | Total time:10 min | Serves: 2)
Ingredients

- 1 12oz can Tuna, in water low sodium
- 1 egg, hard boiled
- ¼ Small Onion, chopped
- 1 Teaspoon Dill Pickle Relish
- 2 Tablespoons Greek Yogurt, Plain
- 1 Teaspoon Mayonnaise
- ½ Teaspoon Garlic Powder
- ½ Teaspoon Black Pepper
- ¼ Teaspoon Salt
- Fresh Bib Lettuce for "wraps"
- Tomatoes for garnish

Instructions

1. Drain water from tuna.
2. Pour drained tuna into a medium bowl and mix with all ingredients except tomato and lettuce.
3. Scoop into lettuce "wraps" and top with sliced tomatoes.

Makes 2 Servings
1 SmartPoints on FreeStyle Plan or FlexPlan

1FS - Cheesy Veggie Egg Scramble

(Prep time:5 min | Cook time:10 min | Total time:15 min | Serves: 6)
Ingredients

- 6 Large Eggs (Cage Free)
- 1 Organic Tomato Diced
- 3 Cups Organic Baby Spinach
- ½ Organic Red Onion Diced
- 1 Clove Garlic Crushed & Minced
- 1 Teaspoon Fresh Cracked Black Pepper
- 1 Teaspoon Kosher Salt
- ½ Cup Organic 2% Sharp Cheddar Cheese (we love Cabot brand)

- 1½ Tablespoons Organic Extra Virgin Olive Oil

Instructions

1. In a large bowl, beat together eggs, black pepper, and salt, set aside.
2. Bring olive oil to temperature in large skillet
3. Add in tomato, spinach, onion, and garlic and sauté for 5-7 minutes or until veggies are cooked through.
4. Pour beaten eggs over vegetables and cook for additional 3-4 minutes stirring occasionally. Cook until egg is set.
5. Remove from heat and sprinkle with cheese.

Makes 6 Servings
1 SmartPoints on FreeStyle Plan or FlexPlan

1FS - Sweet & Sour Turkey Meatballs

Prep time: 5 mins
Cook time: 15 mins
Total time: 20 mins
Serves: 6

Ingredients

- 1 pound 99% Ground Turkey breast or Ground Chicken Breast
- ½ Teaspoon Salt
- 1 Teaspoon Black Pepper
- 1 Teaspoon Onion Powder
- 1 Teaspoon Garlic Powder
- 1 Teaspoon Paprika
- 1 Teaspoon Cumin
- ¼ teriyaki sauce
- ¼ Cup Sugar-Free BBQ Sauce
- ⅛ cup apple cider vinegar
- 1 tablespoon brown sugar twin

Instructions

1. In a large bowl, mix together ground meat and spices (salt, pepper, onion powder, garlic powder, paprika, and cumin). Mix until well blended.
2. In a small bowl, mix together the teriyaki sauce, BBQ sauce, apple cider vinegar, and brown sugar twin.
3. Add ¼ cup of sauce mixture to meat mixture and mix well.

4. Roll meat mixture into 1½" balls. Should make about 12 meatballs
5. Place meatballs on a lined baking sheet (we use silicone baking mats) about 1" apart
6. Bake at 375 degrees for 10 minutes. Turn meatballs, and cook for additional 10 minutes.
7. Remove from oven and toss with sauce until well coated.

WW Information:
Makes 6 servings of 3 meatballs per serving
1 SmartPoint on FreeStyle Plan or Flex Plan

1FS - White Bean Turkey Chili

(Prep time:15 min | Cook time:60 min | Total time:75 min | Serves: 8)
Ingredients
- 2 cups shredded cooked turkey
- ½ cup diced onion
- ½ green pepper, diced
- ½ cup diced celery
- 2 tablespoons olive oil
- 1 tablespoon minced garlic
- 2 cups chicken broth
- 3 cans (15-16 oz.) white beans / great northern beans
- ¼ teaspoon cayenne pepper
- 1 teaspoon ground cumin
- ¾ teaspoon oregano
- ½ teaspoon salt
- ¼ teaspoon ground black pepper
- shredded Parmesan cheese, sour cream, and cilantro for serving if desired

Instructions
1. In a large stock pot or Dutch oven, add onion, green pepper, celery and olive oil. Cook on medium-high heat until onions are translucent and peppers are tender. Stir in garlic.
2. Add chicken broth, beans, and turkey and mix well. Stir in seasonings. Heat to boiling then reduce heat to simmer and cover for 30-60 minutes, stirring occasionally.

3. Heat to boiling then reduce heat to simmer and cover for 30-60 minutes, stirring occasionally.
4. Serve with sour cream, cheese, and cilantro.

Makes 8 Servings (approximately 1 cup each)
1 SmartPoints on FreeStyle Plan or FlexPlan

1FS - Sweet & Sour Meatballs

(Prep time:5 min | Cook time:15 min | Total time:20 min | Serves: 6)
Ingredients

- 1 pound 99% Ground Turkey breast or Ground Chicken Breast
- ½ Teaspoon Salt
- 1 Teaspoon Black Pepper
- 1 Teaspoon Onion Powder
- 1 Teaspoon Garlic Powder
- 1 Teaspoon Paprika
- 1 Teaspoon Cumin
- ¼ teriyaki sauce
- ¼ Cup Sugar-Free BBQ Sauce
- ⅛ cup apple cider vinegar
- 1 tablespoon brown sugar twin

Instructions

1. In a large bowl, mix together ground meat and spices (salt, pepper, onion powder, garlic powder, paprika, and cumin).Mix until well blended.
2. In a small bowl, mix together the teriyaki sauce, BBQ sauce, apple cider vinegar, and brown sugar twin.
3. Add ¼ cup of sauce mixture to meat mixture and mix well.
4. Roll meat mixture into 1½" balls.Should make about 12 meatballs
5. Place meatballs on a lined baking sheet (we use silicone baking mats) about 1" apart
6. Bake at 375 degrees for 10 minutes.Turn meatballs, and cook for additional 10 minutes.
7. Remove from oven and toss with sauce until well coated.

Makes 6 servings of 3 meatballs per serving
1 SmartPoints on FreeStyle Plan or FlexPlan

1FS - Chicken Taco Soup Recipe

Prep time: 5 mins
Cook time: 30 mins
Total time: 35 mins
Serves: 8

Ingredients

- 2 Cups Shredded or Cubed Chicken
- 1 onion, diced
- 1 bell pepper, diced
- 1 poblano pepper, diced
- 2 tomatoes, chopped
- 1 tablespoon garlic, minced
- 6 cups fat free chicken broth
- 1 cup tomato sauce
- 1½ cups kidney beans or pinto beans
- 2 tablespoons taco/fajita seasoning
- 1 tablespoon olive oil

Instructions

1. In a large stockpot, sauté the onion, bell pepper, poblano pepper, and tomato for 5 minutes stirring regularly. You want the vegetables to be tender.
2. Mix in chicken, broth, tomato sauce, garlic, pinto beans, and seasonings.
3. Simmer on medium heat for 30 minutes, stirring occasionally.
4. Serve with preferred garnishes like cheese, sour cream, or tortilla chips.

WW Information:

Makes 8 Servings (approximately 2 cups each)
1 SmartPoint per serving on FreeStyle Plan or FlexPlan

2FS – Tasty Baked Pumpkin Pie Eggroll

Prep time: 15 mins
Cook time: 15 mins
Total time: 30 mins
Serves: 4

Ingredients

- ¾ cup pumpkin puree
- ¼ cup greek yogurt
- 2 Tbsp. Brown sugar
- 1 tsp. pumpkin pie spice
- 4 egg roll wrappers
- Optional:
- fat free Cool-Whip
- Cinnamon for sprinkling
- cooking spray

Instructions

1. Preheat oven to 350 degrees
2. Whisk together pumpkin, yogurt brown sugar, and pumpkin pie spice until well combined.
3. Spread out egg roll wrappers with one point directly to you and one pointing away and place ¼ cup of mixture across the center.
4. Fold up the bottom corner, wet your finger and run it across the edge of all remaining sides.(This acts as a glue)
5. Fold sides inward, pressing the egg roll wrapper together lightly.
6. Tuck and roll the final corner, pressing wrappers well to each other to form a seal, add a touch more water if needed to make sure its sealed, or your filling will leak out.
7. Place eggrolls on a parchment paper lined or non stick sprayed baking sheet (or I use a pizza stone). Coat the tops of your eggrolls lightly with nonstick spray to crisp them up a bit. Bake for 11-13 minutes until crisp and browned.

MAKES 4 SERVINGS – 1 EGG ROLL PER SERVING
2 SMARTPOINTS PER SERVING ON FREESTYLE PLAN OR FLEX PLAN

2FS - Tasty BBQ Apricot Chicken

Prep time: 5 mins, Cook time: 30 mins, Total time: 35 mins
Serves: 6

Ingredients

- 1 pound boneless skinless chicken breasts
- ½ cup sugar-free apricot jam

- ½ cup G Hughes Sugar Free BBQ Sauce
- 2 tablespoons low sodium soy sauce
- 1 teaspoon garlic powder
- 1 teaspoon onion powder
- 1 teaspoon ground ginger

Instructions

1. In a medium bowl, whisk together the jam, bbq sauce, soy sauce, and seasonings.
2. Line baking sheet with foil and place chicken breasts in even layer
3. Pour barbecue sauce over chicken making sure well covered.
4. Bake at 350 degrees for 30 minutes.
5. Remove from oven, and serve with favorite sides.

WW Information:

Makes 6 Servings (approximately 3oz each)
2 SmartPoints per serving on Freestyle or FlexPlan

2FS - Cheesy & Grilled Cream Corn

Prep time: 5 mins
Cook time: 20 mins
Total time: 25 mins
Makes 8 servings Each Serving is approximately ⅓ cup 2 SmartPoints per Serving on FreeStyle Plan or FlexPlan

Ingredients

- 16 oz. bag frozen sweet corn
- ½ cup fat-free mayonnaise
- ¼ cup grated Parmesan cheese
- ½ cup plain non-fat Greek yogurt
- ½-3/4 tsp. cayenne pepper
- ½-3/4 tsp. black pepper

Instructions

1. Combine corn, mayonnaise, Parmesan cheese, Greek yogurt, cayenne pepper, and black pepper in a large bowl stir well until all ingredients are combined thoroughly.
2. Place in grill-safe cooking pan or dish and cover tightly with aluminum foil.

3. Heat on the top shelf of the grill. The bottom is fine if you don't have 2 racks,
4. Cook for 5-7 minutes or until heated through and all ingredients melted.
5. Oven instructions:
6. Preheat oven to 375 degrees and spray pan with nonstick spray.
7. Mix all ingredients together in a large bowl and pour into prepared pan.
8. Bake at 375 for 20 minutes.

2FS - Delicious French Onion Pork

Ingredients:
2 ½ pounds sweet onions, thinly sliced (I use my mandolin slicer.)
2 T. light butter, melted
2 tsp. brown sugar (loosely measured – not packed)
1 T. minced garlic (about 3 cloves)
2 T. all-purpose flour
1 ¾ pounds boneless pork loin
2 packets Lipton Recipe Secrets Onion Soup & Dip Mix
Bread of choice – I used a French baguette, sliced & toasted
Sliced cheese of choice – I used Provolone

Instructions:
Toss the sliced onions in your slow cooker with the melted butter, brown sugar, and garlic until evenly coat onions. Cook on high for at least an hour and a half. Stir in flour and cook 30 minutes more on high. This part can be done the night before, if desired, and refrigerated until the next day.

Place the pork roast on top of the onions and sprinkle in both packets of Lipton Onion Soup & Dip Mix. Reduce heat to low and cook for 8 to 10 hours. No water was needed for mine. It produced plenty of its own juice. If you are leaving it alone to cook all day, you can certainly add half a cup or so of water or beef broth if you're concerned about it getting too dry.

Shred the pork and stir it together with the onions. Serve the onion/pork mixture over toasted bread and top with cheese. Don't forget to put it in an oven-safe pan or skillet. Toasting the cheese under the broiler before serving is well-worth the bit of extra time.

Weight Watchers Info.:
4 ounces of the pork/onion mixture is 2 SmartPoints; same points under the new Freestyle plan.
Don't Forget to calculate your bread & cheese selections.

3FS - Savory Chicken Dump Soup

3 FreeStyle Smart Points per serving (approximately 12 servings / 1 cup each)

Ingredients:
- 1 pound (approx. 3-4) raw skinless boneless chicken thighs
- 1 pkg Trader Joe's frozen Multigrain Blend with Vegetables (if you don't have a TJ's first of all bless your heart.
- Second find another frozen mix with some similar combo to this: cooked grain barley, corn, spelt [wheat], whole rice ermes variety [red], whole rice ribe variety, whole rice-venus variety [black], salt), peas, carrots, water, zucchini, vinegar, extra virgin olive oil, onion, sugar, salt, pepper and totaling no more than 17 SP for the entire bag
- 2 cups (one small package) shredded cabbage
- 1 cup (one small carton fresh or one can) sliced mushrooms any type
- 6 cups water
- 2 tsp dry Italian seasoning

Directions
1. This first part I prep ahead and have on hand in the freezer for easy dumping. If you are anxious to try this right away though there is no need to wait! Just plan a little extra time so your family and friends don't pass out smelling all that yumminess while they stalk you in the kitchen with empty bowls in hand.
2. Add all of the chicken and 1/2 the water to a tall stock pot.

3. Bring everything to a boil for 10 minutes. Reduce to a heavy simmer (not boiling, but bubbling vigorously) and cover loosely with aluminum foil. Let simmer for approximately an hour.
4. Remove one thigh and test with a meat thermometer. If the internal temp is not at least 150 (you want 165 when everything is done!) return and continue simmering for 15 minute intervals until chicken is completely done. If you are making this for prep, remove from heat and allow to cool.
5. Pull chicken apart with two forks to shred or use a hand mixer to "shred" (I haven't used the hand mixer method but I want to try it!).
6. Return to the broth you have just made and then transfer all to a freezer safe container. If you are using immediately return everything to the stock pot and go to the next step.
7. With your stock and shredded chicken in the stock pot, next dump all of the remaining ingredients and stir.
8. Bring back up to a low boil for 10 minutes, then reduce heat and simmer for 30-45 minutes

3FS - Chicken Nuggets with Honey Mustard

Prep time: 5 mins
Cook time: 25 mins
Total time: 30 mins
Serves: 4

Ingredients
- 1 pound boneless skinless chicken breasts
- ½ cup all-purpose flour
- 20 Pretzel Sticks or Mini pretzels
- ¼ cup spicy brown mustard
- ¼ cup skim milk
- 1 tsp. garlic powder
- ½ tsp. black pepper

Instructions
1. Preheat oven to 400 degrees.
2. Put pretzels in a plastic zippered bag and seal. Crush using a rolling pin, heavy glass, or a food processor.

3. Use 3 shallow containers to create your dredging station.
4. Place the flour with pepper and garlic into one. Place the milk and mustard into a second container. Place the crushed pretzels into the final container.
5. Cut chicken into small bite-sized pieces.
6. Dredge chicken in flour, then mustard mixture, and finally pretzel pieces.
7. Place on a baking sheet and bake for 20-23 minutes, until golden brown.

Makes 4 Servings
3 SmartPoints on the FreeStyle or Flex Plans

3FS – Butter Chicken Slow Cook

Prep time: 15 mins
Cook time: 4 hours
Total time: 4 hours 15 mins
Serves: 8

Ingredients
- 1 pound boneless skinless chicken breasts, cut into 1" pieces
- 1 cup unsweetened coconut milk
- 1 cup fat-free plain yogurt
- ½ cup fat-free sour cream
- 2½ tablespoons butter
- 1 cup tomato sauce
- 1 medium tomato diced
- 1 small onion diced
- 2 cloves garlic minced
- 2 teaspoons Garam Masala
- 1 teaspoon ground cumin
- 1 teaspoon ground ginger
- ½ teaspoon chili powder (optional)
- 1 bay leaf
- 1½ teaspoons salt (less if preferred)
- Juice of 1 lemon

Instructions

1. Place chicken in the bottom of your slow cooker. Top with diced onion, garlic, and tomato.
2. Sprinkle with Garam Masala, cumin, ginger, chili powder, and salt.
3. Pour in tomato sauce, unsweetened coconut milk, butter, sour cream, yogurt, and lemon juice.
4. Stir everything until well combined.
5. Add bay leaf.
6. Cook on high heat for 3 hours.
7. Stir well, reduce to low heat and cook additional 1 hour.
8. Serve with rice.

Makes 8 Servings
4 SmartPoints Per Serving (without rice)
2 SmartPoints Per Serving on Freestyle Plan or FlexPlan

3FS – Delicious Apple Cinnamon Muffins

Prep time: 5 mins
Cook time: 18 mins
Total time: 23 mins
Serves: 18

Ingredients
- 1 Sugar-Free Cake Mix (white or yellow)
- 1½ cups Granny Smith apples, chopped (approximately 3 small apples in ¼" dices)
- ½ cup unsweetened applesauce
- 1 small ripe banana
- 1 cup water
- 2 teaspoons ground cinnamon

Instructions
1. Preheat oven to 375 degrees.
2. Spray with nonstick spray or line full sized muffin tins.
3. In a large bowl, mash banana and mix well with applesauce.
4. Mix together dry cake mix and cinnamon in large bowl.
5. Pour mashed banana and applesauce mixture as well as water over dry mixture and lightly mix, but don't completely blend.

6. Add in apples, and mix well.
7. Pour approximately ¼ cup mixture into each muffin tin. This should make enough for 18 muffins.
8. Bake at 375 degrees for 18 minutes or until golden brown and cooked through.
9. These will be moist, but should not be liquid in the center.

Makes 18 Muffins (using full sized muffin tin, but not overfilled muffins)
3 SmartPoints per muffin on FreeStyle and FlexPlan

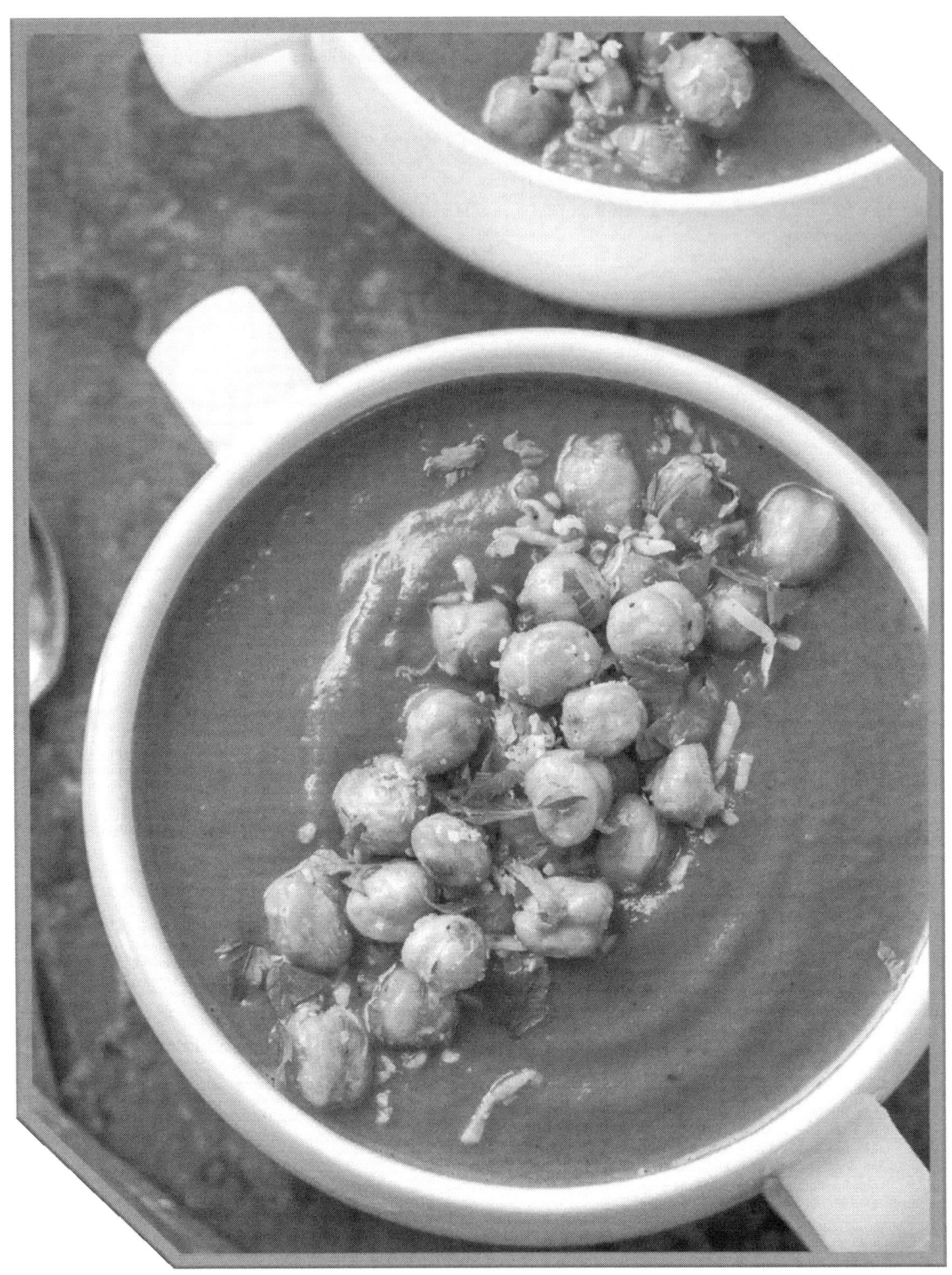

4FS - Simple Taco Salad

Serves: 4
4 SmartPoints™

Ingredients:

½ pound ground beef
½ teaspoon salt
1 teaspoon black pepper
½ teaspoon garlic powder
1 teaspoon cumin
½ cup fresh corn kernels
1 cup tomatoes, cubed
1 avocado, cubed
5 cups lettuce or salad mix, chopped
Fresh lime quarters for garnish, optional

Directions:

1. Place the ground beef in a skillet over medium heat.

2. Cook until the meat is completely browned, approximately 7-10 minutes. Drain off any excess fat. Season the meat with salt, black pepper, garlic powder, and cumin.

3. In a bowl, combine the cooked ground beef, fresh corn kernels, tomatoes, avocado and chopped lettuce. Toss gently to mix.

4. Serve the salad with fresh lime wedges for dressing the salad, if desired.

Nutritional Information:

Calories 258, Total Fat 18.9 g, Saturated Fat 5.7 g, Total Carbohydrate 11.2 g, Dietary Fiber 5.1 g, Sugars 0.8 g, Protein 13.0 g

4FS - Fruit & Blue Cheese Tossed Salad

Serves: 4
4 SmartPoints™

Ingredients:

4 tablespoons balsamic vinegar
4 teaspoons maple syrup
Salt to taste
2 tablespoons olive oil

6 cups mixed baby spinach leaves

2 medium pears, sliced

¼ cup blue cheese, chopped

1 tablespoon pine nuts (optional)

Directions:

1. Mix the vinegar, maple syrup, salt, and olive oil in a small bowl. Mix well until everything has combined properly.

2. Mix the baby spinach, lettuce, and pears in a large bowl and sprinkle the salad with the dressing. Toss to coat.

3. Spread the blue cheese and the pine nuts on top of the salad. Serve immediately.

Nutritional Information:

Calories 149, Total Fat 9.7 g, Saturated Fat 2.6 g, Total Carbohydrate 15.0 g, Dietary Fiber 3.6 g, Sugars 7.0 g, Protein 3.4 g

4FS - Chicken and Spinach Rings

Serves: 8

4 SmartPoints™

Ingredients:

5 ounces grilled chicken, cut in strips

1 cup baby spinach, fresh

1 (8 ounce) can crescent roll dough (reduced fat)

4 tablespoons whipped cream cheese (reduced fat), softened

⅓ Cup Mexican blend cheese (reduced fat), shredded

Spices of your choice

Directions:

1. Preheat the oven to 375°F.

2. Arrange the crescent roll dough, unrolled, on an ungreased baking sheet. Spread the cream cheese on each, and then season with your favorite spices.

3. Place the spinach on top of the cream cheese and lay on the grilled chicken strips. Sprinkle with the Mexican blend cheese. Make the rings by pulling

the ends of each crescent roll up and wrapping it around the filling. Tuck them so they retain the shape.

4. Bake for 14 minutes, or until the crescent rolls become golden brown.

Nutritional Information:
Calories 142, Total Fat 5.0 g, Saturated Fat 2.0 g, Total Carbohydrate 16.0 g, Dietary Fiber 1.0 g, Sugars 1.0 g, Protein 8.0 g

4FS - Bruschetta Topped Balsamic Chicken

Yield: 4 SERVINGS

INGREDIENTS:

- 4 (6 oz.) raw boneless skinless chicken breasts or cutlets
- Salt and pepper, to taste
- ½ teaspoon dried oregano
- 2 teaspoons olive oil, divided
- ¾ cup balsamic vinegar
- 2 tablespoons sugar
- ¼ teaspoon salt
- 1 cup chopped cherry or grape tomatoes
- 1-2 tablespoons of sliced fresh basil
- 1 teaspoon minced garlic (or more to taste)

DIRECTIONS:

1. Pre-heat the oven to 400 degrees. Place the chicken breasts on a cutting board and if necessary, pound with a meat mallet to ensure an even thickness.
2. Sprinkle each breast with salt, pepper and oregano on each side.
3. Pour 1 ½ teaspoons of olive oil into a large skillet and bring over medium-high heat.
4. Place the breasts in the pan in a single layer and cook for 1-2 minutes on each side to lightly brown the outside of the chicken.
5. Mist a baking sheet with cooking spray and place the chicken breasts onto the sheet. Cover with aluminum foil and bake for 15 minutes.
6. While the chicken is baking, combine the balsamic vinegar, sugar and salt in a small saucepan and stir to combine. Bring to a boil over medium-high heat and then reduce the heat to medium low. Simmer for 10-15 minutes until the mixture has reduced and thickened and will coat the back of a spoon. Split the balsamic glaze into two small dishes.

7. When the chicken comes out of the oven, discard any extra liquid produced by the chicken. Use a pastry brush to brush the glaze from one of the dishes onto the chicken breasts. Place the baking sheet of chicken back in the oven, uncovered this time, for 5-10 minutes until the chicken is cooked through. Wash your pastry brush thoroughly.
8. Combine the chopped tomatoes, sliced basil, minced garlic and the remaining ½ teaspoon of olive oil in a bowl and add salt and pepper to taste. Stir to combine.
9. When the chicken breasts are done cooking, brush the second dish of balsamic glaze over the chicken breasts. Serve each breast topped with ¼ cup of the bruschetta tomato mixture.

WEIGHT WATCHERS FREESTYLE SMARTPOINTS:
4 per serving NUTRITION INFORMATION:
293 calories, 18 g carbs, 17 g sugars, 7 g fat, 1 g saturated fat, 39 g protein, 1 g fiber .

5FS - Ham & Apricot Dijon Glaze

5 Free Style Smart Points 145 calories
TOTAL TIME: 5 hours
INGREDIENTS:
- 1 (6 to 7 pound) Hickory smoked fully cooked spiral cut ham
- 5 tbsp. apricot preserves
- 2 tablespoons Dijon mustard

DIRECTIONS:
1. Make the glaze: Whisk 4 tablespoons of preserves and mustard together.
2. Place the ham in a 6-quart or larger slow cooker, making sure you can put the lid on. You may have to turn the ham on its side if your ham is too large.
3. Brush the glaze over the ham. Cover and cook on the LOW setting for 4 to 5 hours. Brush the remaining tablespoon of preserves over the ham the 30 minutes.

NUTRITION INFORMATION
Yield: 16, Serving Size: 3 ounces
- Amount Per Serving:
Smart Points: 5, Calories: 145, Total Fat: 7g, Saturated Fat: 1.5g

Carbohydrates: 12g, Fiber: 0g, Sugar: 11g, Protein: 15g

5FS – Fresh & Freestyle Egg Salad

Serves: 4
5 SmartPoints™
Ingredients:
4 large eggs
2 large egg whites
2 tablespoon mayonnaise (reduced-calorie)
1 teaspoon fresh dill, shopped
2 tablespoon fresh chives, chopped
$\frac{1}{2}$ teaspoon Dijon mustard
½ teaspoon table salt or to taste
¼ teaspoon black pepper, freshly ground
Directions:

1. Place all 6 eggs in a saucepan and add water to cover.

2. Cover the saucepan with a lid and set it over high heat to boil. Boil for about 10 minutes, and drain the water. Place the eggs in ice water to cool so you'll be able to handle them. When the eggs are cool, remove and discard the shells from all the 6 eggs and the yolks of 2 eggs, keeping the egg whites.

3. Cut the 4 whole eggs and the 2 egg whites into ½-inch pieces with a knife or an egg slicer. Transfer the cut eggs to a medium bowl and add the mayonnaise, dill, chives, mustard, salt and pepper. Mix all the ingredients together until they have blended well. Serve and enjoy.

Nutritional Information:
Calories 106, Total Fat 7.3 g, Saturated Fat 1.9 g, Total Carbohydrate 1.3 g, Dietary Fiber 0.1 g, Sugars 1.0 g, Protein 8.2 g

5FS - Chicken Club Salad

Serves: 4
5 SmartPoints™
Ingredients:
8 cups mixed dark salad greens
1 pound chicken, cooked and sliced

½ cup bacon, cooked and diced

2 cups heirloom tomatoes, cut into wedges

½ cup fat free ranch dressing

Directions:

1. Place the salad greens in a bowl and add the fat free ranch dressing. Toss to coat.

2. Next, add the chicken, bacon, and tomatoes. Toss to mix.

3. Serve immediately, or cover and refrigerate for up to two hours before serving.

Nutritional Information:

Calories 215, Total Fat 4.6 g, Saturated Fat 1.3 g, Total Carbohydrate 11.0 g, Dietary Fiber 1.3 g, Sugars 5.2 g, Protein 28.1 g

5FS - Mushroom Egg Drop Soup

Serves: 4

5 SmartPoints™

Ingredients:

4 cups chicken stock

5 wonton wrappers

1 cup oyster mushrooms, thinly sliced

2 eggs, beaten

1 teaspoon soy sauce

½ teaspoon salt

1 teaspoon white pepper

Scallions, sliced for garnish (optional)

Lime slices for garnish (optional)

Directions:

1. Place the chicken stock in a soup pan and bring it to a boil over medium-high heat. Once the stock comes to a boil, reduce the heat to medium low.

2. While the stock is coming to a boil, lay the wonton wrappers out on the counter and slice them into ½-inch thick pieces.

3. Add the mushrooms and sliced wonton wrappers to the chicken stock and cook for 1-2 minutes.

4. In a bowl, combine the beaten eggs, soy sauce, salt, and white pepper. Whisk together.

5. Slowly pour the egg mixture into the soup, whisking constantly to create thin strips of cooked egg throughout the soup. Cook for an additional 1-2 minutes.

6. Remove the soup from the heat and serve warm, garnished with scallions and lime, if desired.

Nutritional Information:
Calories 151, Total Fat 5.3 g, Saturated Fat 1.6 g, Total Carbohydrate 15.1 g, Dietary Fiber 0.5 g, Sugars 3.9 g, Protein 10.4 g a

Makes 8 servings.

One serving is 1-1/2 cups soup.

5 WW FreeStyle SP per serving.

INGREDIENTS

- Cooking spray
- 1 onion, chopped
- 3-4 carrots, sliced or chopped
- 1 cup green beans, cut
- 2 minced garlic cloves
- 1 (24 ounce) package Jennie-O Italian style turkey meatballs
- 2 (14.5 ounce) cans beef or vegetable broth
- 2 (14.5 ounce) diced or Italian stewed tomatoes
- 1-1/2 cups frozen corn
- 1 teaspoon oregano
- 1 teaspoon parsley
- ½ teaspoon basil

INSTRUCTIONS

1. Spray large saucepan or instant pot with cooking spray.
2. Add onions, carrots, green beans and garlic and cook over medium heat 2-3 minutes.
3. Mix in remaining ingredients.
4. If cooking on a stovetop, cover and cook over medium-low heat for 20 minutes, or until meatballs are heated through.
5. -OR-
6. If using an instant pot, press the "soup" button and cook on high pressure for 15 minutes. Vent to release pressure once cooked.
7. -OR-
8. Cook in a slow cooker for 5-6 hours on LOW.
9. Serve warm.
10. Refrigerate or freeze leftovers.

Nutrition Information

- Serves: 8 servings
- Serving size: 1-1/2 cup soup

Calories: 285, Fat: 13 g, Saturated fat: 4 g, Carbohydrates: 21 g
Sugar: 9 g, Protein: 19 g

Serves: 4
Ingredients

- 1 cup low sodium chicken broth (or vegetable broth if you prefer)
- 1 14 oz. can tomato puree
- 1 cup skim milk
- 4-5 leaves fresh basil
- 3 tsp. olive oil
- 1 stalk celery
- ½ cup onions
- 1 Tbsp. cornstarch
- 1-2 cloves garlic, crushed.
- pepper to taste

Instructions

1. Rough chop onions and celery, transfer them to a food processor or chopper and puree until fine.
2. Heat olive oil in a large pan over medium heat.
3. Add onion and celery mix to pan and sauté until they begin to become translucent.
4. Reduce heat to low and stir in garlic, pepper, chicken stock, and tomato puree, and cornstarch-simmer on low for 5 minutes.
5. Whisk in tomato puree and milk, top with basil leaves, simmer for an additional 10 minutes.
6. Serve topped with a dollop of Greek yogurt or a fresh chopped basil.
7. This makes approximately 4 -1/2 cup servings

Makes 2 large servings
5 SmartPoints per serving on FreeStyle Plan, and Flex Plan

5FS - Sticky Buffalo Chicken Tenders

Prep time: 10 mins, Cook time: 15 mins, Total time: 25 mins

Ingredients

- 1 pound boneless skinless chicken breasts, pounded to ½" thickness
- ¼ cup flour
- 3 eggs
- 1 cup Italian Seasoned Panko breadcrumbs
- ½ cup brown sugar
- ⅓ cup Frank's Red Hot Sauce
- ½ teaspoon Garlic Powder
- 3 tablespoons water

Instructions

1. Preheat oven to 425 degrees and spray a baking sheet with non-stick cooking spray or line with silicone baking mats.
2. Cut boneless skinless chicken breasts into strips or chunks (we find chunks hold coating better).
3. Add the chicken into a large Ziploc bag that contains just the flour. Shake to coat.
4. Place Panko breadcrumbs into a shallow bowl. In another shallow bowl, whisk eggs until combined well.
5. Dip flour coated chicken into eggs, then into Panko breadcrumbs to coat.
6. Place coated chicken on the prepared baking sheet. Spray tops with non-stick cooking spray.
7. Bake for 15 minutes for nuggets or 20 minutes for strips or until chicken is browned and cooked through.
8. While chicken is in the oven, you will make your sauce mixture.
9. In a medium saucepan, bring the brown sugar, garlic powder, water and Frank's red hot sauce to a boil. Remove from heat and stir well.
10. When chicken is cooked through, remove from the oven and toss with sauce. This will just coat the chicken.

Makes 6 Servings

5 SmartPoints per Serving on FreeStyle or Flex Plan

5FS - Garlic Roasted Garbanzo Beans

Prep time: 5 mins, Cook time: 45 mins, Total time: 50 mins

Ingredients

- 1 can garbanzo beans (chickpeas)
- 1 tablespoon olive oil
- 1 teaspoon salt
- 1 teaspoon garlic powder
- ½ teaspoon paprika

Instructions

1. Preheat oven to 375° Fahrenheit.
2. Line a baking sheet with a silicone baking mat or parchment paper.
3. Drain and rinse the garbanzo beans.
4. Pat garbanzo beans dry, pour into a large bowl.
5. Toss with olive oil, salt, garlic powder, and paprika until all are well coated.
6. Spread evenly over baking sheet.
7. Bake at 375° for 20 minutes. Turn chickpeas so they are evenly roasted (use a spatula to flip them or simply stir around but make sure they are in an even layer).
8. Place back in the oven at 375° for additional 25 minutes.
9. Allow the roasted garbanzo beans to cool before storing in an airtight container for snacking.

Makes approximately 3 servings

5 SmartPoints per 1/2 cup on FreeStyle, and Flex Plan

5FS - Roasted Sweet Potato Side Dish

Prep time: 5 mins, Cook time: 25 mins, Total time: 30 mins

Ingredients

- 2 Medium Sweet Potatoes
- ½ teaspoon salt
- Non-Stick Cooking Spray

Instructions

1. Preheat oven to 400 degrees.
2. Line baking sheet with silicone baking mat or spray with non-stick spray.
3. Clean sweet potatoes, and peel if desired. We usually leave the skin intact. Remove any blemishes or eyes if needed.
4. Slice sweet potatoes into ¼" thick medallions
5. Place sweet potatoes in a single layer on prepared baking sheet.
6. Sprinkle the tops lightly with salt.
7. Bake at 400 degrees for 15 minutes. Turn sweet potato medallions over and bake additional 10 minutes.

This recipe makes 4 servings.

Each serving is approximately 1/2 sweet potato.

5 SmartPoints per serving on FreeStyle Plan or Flex Plan

5FS - Chicken Marsala MeatBall

5 Free Style Smart Points 248 calories

TOTAL TIME: 30 minutes

INGREDIENTS:

- 8 ounces sliced cremini mushrooms, divided
- 1 pound 93% lean ground chicken
- 1/3 cup whole wheat seasoned or gluten-free bread crumbs
- 1/4 cup grated Pecorino cheese
- 1 large egg, beaten
- 3 garlic cloves, minced
- 2 tablespoons chopped fresh parsley, plus more for garnish
- 1 teaspoon Kosher salt
- Freshly ground black pepper
- 1/2 tablespoon all-purpose flour
- 1/2 tablespoon unsalted butter
- 1/4 cup finely chopped shallots
- 3 ounces sliced shiitake mushrooms
- 1/3 cup Marsala wine
- 3/4 cup reduced sodium chicken broth

DIRECTIONS:

1. Preheat the oven to 400F.
2. Finely chop half of the Cremini mushrooms and transfer to a medium bowl with the ground chicken, breadcrumbs, Pecorino, egg, 1 clove of the minced garlic, parsley, 1 teaspoon kosher salt and black pepper, to taste.
3. Gently shape into 25 small meatballs, bake 15 to 18 minutes, until golden.
4. In a small bowl whisk the flour with the Marsala wine and broth.
5. Heat a large skillet on medium heat.
6. Add the butter, garlic and shallots and cook until soft and golden, about 2 minutes.
7. Add the mushrooms, season with 1/8 teaspoon salt and a pinch of black pepper, and cook, stirring occasionally, until golden, about 5 minutes.
8. Return the meatballs to the pot, pour the Marsala wine mixture over the meatballs, cover and cook 10 minutes.

9. Garnish with parsley.

NUTRITION INFORMATION

Yield: 5 servings, Serving Size: 5 meatballs with mushrooms

- Amount Per Serving:

Smart Points: 5, Calories: 248, Total Fat: 4g, Saturated Fat: 4g

Carbohydrates: 13g, Fiber: 1.5g, Sugar: 4.5g, Protein: 21g

5FS - Asparagus and Chicken Salad

Serves: 4

5 SmartPoints™

Ingredients:

1 ½ pounds fresh asparagus, trimmed

12 endive leaves, trimmed

2 cups chicken, cooked and sliced

½ teaspoon salt, optional

½ teaspoon black pepper, optional

¼ cup stilton cheese crumbles

½ lemon, zested and juiced

Directions:

1. Place the asparagus spears in a skillet and add just enough water to cover.

2. Turn the heat on to medium-high and bring the water to a boil. Cover, reduce the heat to low and simmer for approximately 5 minutes, or until the asparagus is firm tender.

3. Remove the asparagus from the pan and immediately place it in a bowl of cold water for 1 minute.

4. Remove the asparagus from the water, drain well and set aside.

5. Arrange 3 endive leaves on each plate, topped with the sliced chicken.

6. Season with salt and pepper, if desired.

7. Next, sprinkle on the stilton cheese crumbles and top with the asparagus.

8. Drizzle with lemon juice to your liking and garnish with lemon zest before serving.

Nutritional Information:
Calories 181, Total Fat 7.0 g, Saturated Fat 4.0 g, Total Carbohydrate 10.4 g, Dietary Fiber 6.8 g, Sugars 0.3 g, Protein 21.0 g

6FS - Roasted Caprese Salad Chicken

Serves: 4
6 SmartPoints™

Ingredients:

4 cups heirloom grape tomatoes, halved
1 ½ tablespoons olive oil
1 teaspoon salt, divided
1 teaspoon black pepper, divided
1 pound boneless, skinless chicken breast, cooked and sliced
1 cup fresh mozzarella bocconcini
½ cup fresh basil, torn
1 tablespoon balsamic vinegar

Directions:

1. Preheat the oven to 400°F and line a baking sheet with parchment paper or aluminum foil.

2. Wash the grape tomatoes and cut each in half.

3. Drizzle the olive oil over the tomatoes and season with half a teaspoon each of salt and black pepper. Toss to mix.

4. Spread the tomatoes out on the baking sheet and place in the oven. Cook for 10-12 minutes. Remove from the oven and allow to cool slightly.

5. Place the tomatoes in a bowl and combine them with the chicken, fresh mozzarella, and basil. Drizzle the salad with the balsamic vinegar and season with the remaining salt and black pepper. Toss gently.

6. Serve immediately, or cover and refrigerate for 30 minutes before serving.

Nutritional Information:
Calories 276, Total Fat 14.1 g, Saturated Fat 5.5 g, Total Carbohydrate 3.5 g, Dietary Fiber 0.0 g, Sugars 1.5 g, Protein 30.7 g

6FS - Raspberry Chicken Salad

Serves: 4
6 SmartPoints™
Ingredients:
6 cup mixed greens (arugula, endive, spinach, etc.)
2 cups cooked chicken, shredded or cubed
¼ cup walnuts, chopped
1 cup fresh raspberries
½ cup feta cheese
Directions:

1. Thoroughly rinse the greens and combine them in a bowl. Toss to mix.

2. Add the chicken and walnuts to the bowl and toss again.

3. At this point, you can either keep all of the ingredients in the large bowl for serving or transfer the salad to individual serving plates.

4. Top the salad with fresh raspberries and crumbled feta cheese.

5. Serve immediately while the greens are still crisp.

Nutritional Information:
Calories 197, Total Fat 10.7 g, Saturated Fat 3.7 g, Total Carbohydrate 5.4 g, Dietary Fiber 4.1 g, Sugars 0.9 g, Protein 17.7 g

6FS - Roasted Cauliflower Soup

Serves: 6, 6 SmartPoints™
Ingredients:
8 cups cauliflower florets (approximately one large head)   ½ cup pancetta, diced
1 cup yellow onion, sliced
1 cup fennel bulb, sliced
2 tablespoons olive oil
2 teaspoons fresh rosemary, chopped
½ teaspoon nutmeg
1 teaspoon salt
1 teaspoon black pepper
6 cups vegetable stock

Directions:

1. Preheat the oven to 450°F and line a baking sheet with aluminum foil.

2. In a bowl, toss together the cauliflower, onion, and fennel. Drizzle the vegetables with olive oil and season with rosemary, nutmeg, salt, and black pepper. Toss to mix.

3. Spread the vegetables out on a baking sheet and place them in the oven. Bake for 15 minutes.

4. While the vegetables are roasting, bring the vegetable stock to a boil in a soup pot over medium high heat.

5. Place the pancetta in a small skillet over medium heat, and cook for 3-5 minutes, stirring frequently, until lightly crispy.

6. Remove the vegetables from the oven and carefully transfer to the boiling vegetable stock. Cover, reduce the heat to low and simmer for 10-14 minutes.

7. Working in batches, transfer the soup to a blender or food processor and puree before adding the soup back to the pot. Continue with the remaining soup until the desired consistency has been reached.

8. Serve warm, garnished with crispy pancetta.

Nutritional Information:
Calories 196, Total Fat 8.2 g, Saturated Fat 2.0 g, Total Carbohydrate 25.8 g, Dietary Fiber 9.4 g, Sugars 3.8 g, Protein 8.9 g

7FS - Apple Cheddar Turkey Wraps

Yield: 1 WRAP

INGREDIENTS:

- 1 Flatout Light Original Flatbread
- 1-2 leaves green leaf lettuce, torn
- 2 oz. thinly sliced deli turkey
- 1 oz. sliced 50% reduced fat sharp cheddar cheese
- 1 ½ teaspoons apple cider vinegar
- ½ teaspoon canola oil
- ½ teaspoon honey
- A pinch of salt and pepper
- ¼ cup matchstick-sliced apple pieces (slice apple into thin, short sticks)
- 1/3 cup coleslaw mix (just the shredded veggies, undressed)

DIRECTIONS:

1. Lay the Flatout flatbread on a clean, dry surface and lay the torn lettuce down the center of the flatbread going the long way (starting at the rounded end and spreading down the length of the flatbread to the other rounded end). You can leave a bit of space at each end as you'll be folding them over, and you do not need to cover the whole flatbread, just an area down the middle. Top the lettuce with the sliced deli turkey and the cheddar cheese. *Make sure to leave an inch or so of room at each end.*

2. In a small mixing bowl, combine the vinegar, oil, honey, salt and pepper and stir until well combined. Add the apples and coleslaw and stir to coat. Lay the apple/coleslaw mixture on top of the other ingredients layered on the wrap.

3. Fold in the rounded ends of the flatbread over the filling. Then fold one of the long edges over the filling and continue to roll until the wrap is completely rolled up. Cut in half and serve.

WEIGHT WATCHERS FREESTYLE SMARTPOINTS:

7 per wrap (SP *calculated using the recipe builder on weightwatchers.com)*

NUTRITION INFORMATION:
277 calories, 26 g carbs, 8 g sugars, 9 g fat, 3 g saturated fat, 28 g protein, 10 g fiber

7FS - Sweet Potato Chili

Serves: 4

7 SmartPoints™

Ingredients: 2 teaspoons olive oil

1 cup red onion, diced

4 cups sweet potatoes, peeled and cut into small cubes

1 teaspoon salt

1 teaspoon coarse ground black pepper

1 tablespoon chili powder

½ teaspoon cinnamon

2 cups black beans, cooked or canned

4 cups vegetable stock

2 cups fresh or jarred salsa

Fresh cilantro for garnish (optional)

Directions:

1. Place the olive oil in a large saucepan or stock pot over medium heat.

2. Add the onions and sauté for 3 minutes.

3. Add the sweet potatoes, salt, black pepper, chili powder and cinnamon. Cook, stirring frequently, for 3 minutes.

4. Next add the remaining ingredients including the black beans, vegetable stock, and salsa. Mix well.

5. Increase the heat to medium high and cook until the liquid begins to boil. Cover and reduce the heat to low. Simmer for 20 minutes, or until the sweet potatoes are tender.

6. Serve warm, garnished with fresh cilantro, if desired.

Nutritional Information:

Calories 324, Total Fat 3.7 g, Saturated Fat 0.6 g, Total Carbohydrate 71.1 g, Dietary Fiber 16.3 g, Sugars 2.5 g, Protein 15.7 g

Yield: 8 PIECES

INGREDIENTS:

- 8 uncooked lasagna noodles
- 15 oz. can tomato sauce
- 1 cup pizza sauce
- ½ teaspoon Italian seasoning
- 1 lb. uncooked hot Italian poultry sausage, casings removed if present (I used Wegmans patties, you can use chicken or turkey sausage)
- 2 oz. turkey pepperoni, chopped (reserve 8 slices un-chopped for topping)
- 1 (15 oz.) container fat free Ricotta cheese
- 1 (10 oz.) package frozen chopped spinach, thawed and squeezed until dry
- 1 large egg
- 2 oz. 2% shredded Mozzarella cheese

DIRECTIONS:

1. Pre-heat the oven to 350. Lightly mist a 9×13 baking dish with cooking spray and set aside.
2. Boil and salt a large pot of water and cook lasagna noodles according to package instructions. Drain and rinse with cold water. Lay noodles flat on a clean dry surface and set aside.
3. In a mixing bowl, combine the tomato sauce, pizza sauce and Italian seasoning and stir together. Set aside.
4. Place the sausage in a large skillet over medium heat and cook until browned, breaking the meat up into small pieces as it cooks. When the sausage is cooked through, add the chopped pepperoni and 1/3 cup of the tomato sauce mixture and stir to combine. Remove from heat.

5. In a mixing bowl, combine the ricotta cheese, spinach and egg and stir until well combined. Spoon 1/3 cup of the cheese mixture onto each lasagna noodle and spread across the surface leaving a little room (about ½") at the far end with no toppings. Top the cheese layer on each noodle with the meat mixture from step four, evenly dividing the meat between the noodles. Starting with one end (not the one with space at the end), roll the noodle over the filling until it becomes a complete roll. Repeat with all noodles.

6. Spoon ½ cup of the tomato sauce mixture into the prepared baking dish and spread across the bottom. Place the lasagna rolls seam down in the dish and spoon or pour the remaining sauce over top. Sprinkle the Mozzarella over the top of the rolls and place a pepperoni on each one. Cover the dish with aluminum foil and bake for 40 minutes.

WEIGHT WATCHERS FREESTYLE SMARTPOINTS:

7 per serving (*SP calculated using the recipe builder on weightwatchers.com*)

NUTRITION INFORMATION:

289 calories, 31 g carbs, 9 g sugars, 8 g fat, 2 g saturated fat, 24 g protein, 4 g fiber

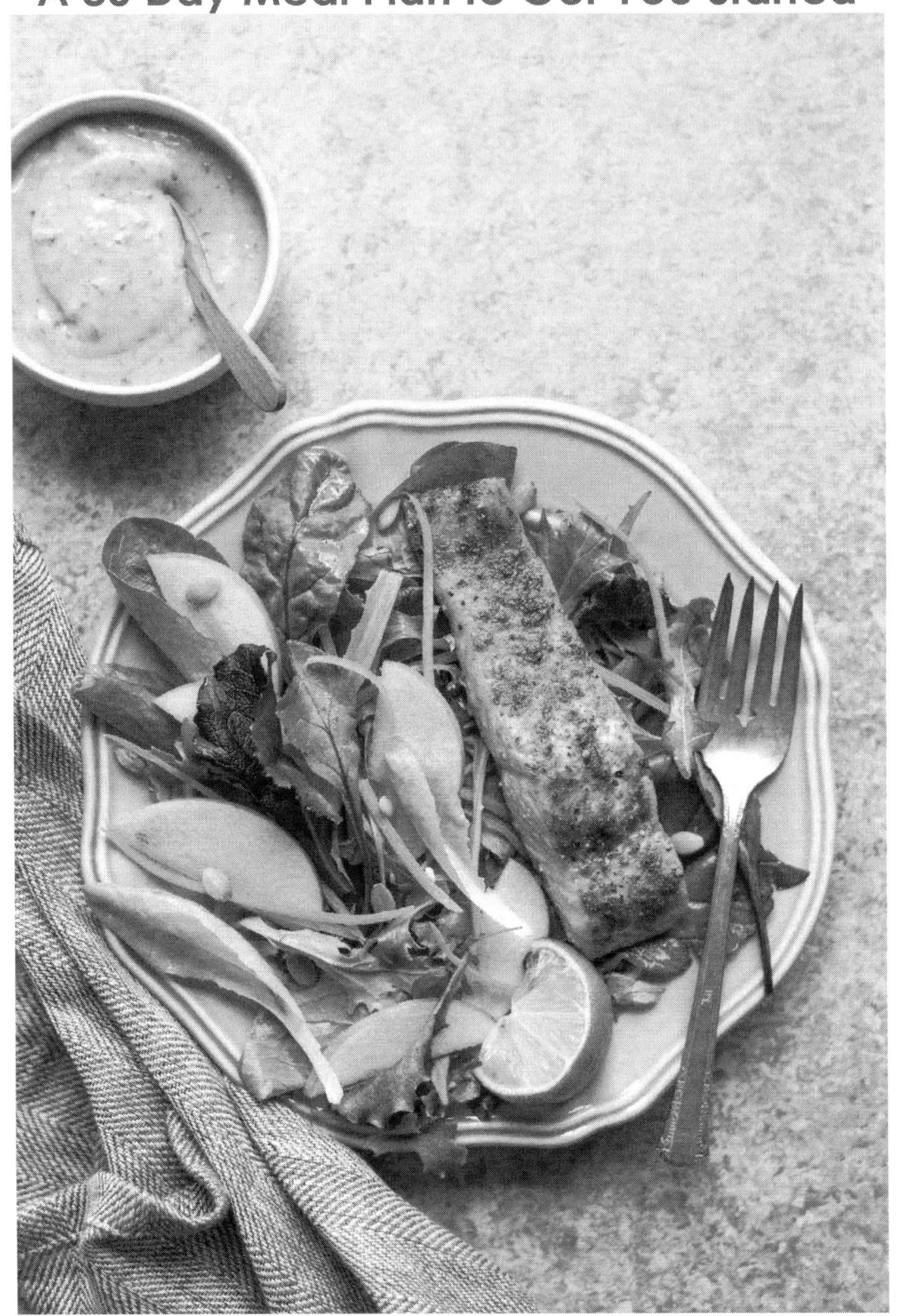

Sometimes one of the hardest things that you will need to do when it comes to getting started on a new meal plan is figure out what meals you would like to cook. There are so many meals out there, but learning which ones belong to your new diet plan and will not make you go over our daily limit can be kind of intimidating in the beginning.

In this chapter, we provide you with a 30-day meal plan that you can follow. There are lots of tasty recipes that you can try and you can find the recipes for all of them inside this guidebook. Whether you are looking for something light on the run or something that is a bit heartier for at night, you are sure to find many recipes that you can love on this list.

So try a few of them out, or use this as your meal planner, and get ready to find out just how great Weight Watchers can be and just how much weight you can lose.

—

Day One:	Breakfast: Pancakes = 6 Lunch: Creamy Pesto Pasta = 7 Dinner: Spinach and Chicken Casserole = 4 Total Points: 17 Points
Day Two:	Breakfast: Healthy Morning Cookies = 2 Lunch: BBQ Pork Sandwich = 5 Dinner: Vegetable Quesadilla = 9 Total Points: 16 Points
Day Three:	Breakfast: Cinnamon Rolls = 6 Lunch: Italian Chicken = 5 Dinner: Veggie Pork Chops = 6 Total Points: 17 Points
Day Four:	Breakfast Mushroom and Spinach Quchie = 3 Lunch: Baked Tortellini = 6 Dinner: Cheese Tuna Sandwich = 10 : Total Points: 19 Points
Day Five:	Breakfast: Apple Muffin: 7 Lunch: Cheesy Mushrooms = 2 Dinner: Cheeseburger Soup = 9 : Total Points:17 Points
Day Six	Breakfast: Potato and Cheese Casserole = 7 Lunch: Baked Burrito = 6 Dinner: Beef Chili = 3 : Total Points: 15 Points

Day Seven	Breakfast: Crispy Apple Surprise = 11 Lunch: Veggie Soup = 1 Dinner: Cilantro Lime Shrimp = 3 Total Points: 15 Points
Day Eight:	Breakfast: Breakfast Jelly Pudding = 11 Lunch: Veggie Soup = 1 Dinner: Spinach and Chicken Crescents = 4 : Total Points:16 Points
Day Nine	Pumpkin Muffins = 4 Lunch: Italian Bread and Tuna Salad = 10 Dinner: Cheesy Chicken Cops = 3 : Total Points:17 Points
Day Ten:	Breakfast: Blackberry and Peach Smoothie = 9 Lunch: Cheeseburger Soup = 7 Dinner Cilantro Lime Shrimp = 3 : Total Points: 19 Points
Day eleven:	Breakfast: Morning Burritos = 9 Lunch: Pasta Veggies = 5 Dinner:Jalapeno Chicken = 4 : Total Points: 18 Points
Day Twelve	Breakfast Souffle = 3 Lunch: Turkey and Cheese Sandwich = 10 Dinner: Jalapeno Chicken = 4 : Total Points: 17 Points

Day thirteen	Breakfast: Breakfast Bars = 6 Lunch: Creamy Pesto Pasta = 7 Dinner: Honey Salmon = 4 : Total Points:17 Points
Day Fourteen	Breakfast: French Toast = 3 Lunch: Baked Fish = 5 Dinner: Mexican Casserole = 8 : Total Points: 16 Points
Day fifteen:	Breakfast: Cheese and Ham Omelet = 6 Lunch: Beef Ziti Bake = 7 Dinner: Cheesy Chicken Chops = 3 : Total Points:16 Points
Day sixteen:	Breakfast: Spiced Honey Cake = 7 Lunch: Chicken Salad = 4 Diner: Veggie Pork Chops = 6 : Total Points: 17 Points
Day seventeen	Breakfast: Blueberry Muffins = 5 Lunch:: BBQ Pork Sandwich = 5 Dinner: Steak and Mashed Potatoes = 9 : Total Points: 18 Pointes
Day eighteen	Breakfast: Yogurt Fluff = 2 Lunch: Baked Fish = 5 Dinner: Pita Bread Pizza =9 : Total Points: 16 Points
Day nineteen	Breakfast: Pancakes = 6 Lunch: Bacon Wraps = 8 Dinner: Egg Salad = 4 : Total Points: 19 Points

Day twenty	Breakfast: Healthy Morning Cookies = 2 Lunch: Beef Burgers = 4 Dinner: Roast Beef with Veggies = 9 : Total Points: 14 Points
Day twenty-one	Breakfast: Cinnamon Rolls = 6 Lunch: Cheesy Mushrooms = 2 Dinner: Cheese and Tuna Sandwich = 10 : Total Points: 18 Points
Day twenty-two	Breakfast: Mushroom and Spinach Quiche = 3 Lunch: Beef Ziti Bake = 7 Dinner: Vegetable Quesadilla = 9 : Total Points 19 Points
Day twenty-three	Breakfast: Apple Muffin = 7 Lunch: Chicken Salad = 4 Dinner: Chicken Thai Wrap =2 : Total Points: 13 Points
Day twenty-four	Breakfast: Potato and Cheese Casserole = 7 Lunch: Bacon wrap = 8 Dinner: Beef Chili = 2 : Total Points: 19 Points
Day twenty-five	Breakfast: Pumpkin Muffins = 4 Lunch: Italian Bread with Tuna Salad = 10 Dinner: Cola Chicken = 5 Total Points 19 Points

Day twenty-six	Breakfast: Blackberry and Peach Smoothie = 9 Lunch: Beef Burgers = 4 Dinner: Mushroom Steak = 5 : Total Points: 18 Points
Day twenty-seven	Breakfast: Morning Burritos = 9 Lunch: Pasta Veggies = 5 Dinner: Beef Chili = 2 Total Points 18 Points
Day twenty0eght	Breakfast: Breakfast Souffle = 3 Lunch: Baked Burrito = 6 Dinner: Baked Chicken = 10 : Total Points:19 Points
Day twenty-nine	Breakfast: Breakfast Bars = 6 Lunch: Baked Tortellini = 6 Dinner: Potato Soup = 4 Total Points: 18 Points
Day thirty	Breakfast: French Toast = 3 Lunch: Italian Chicken = 5 Dinner: Chicken Dumplings = 9 Total Points = 17 Points

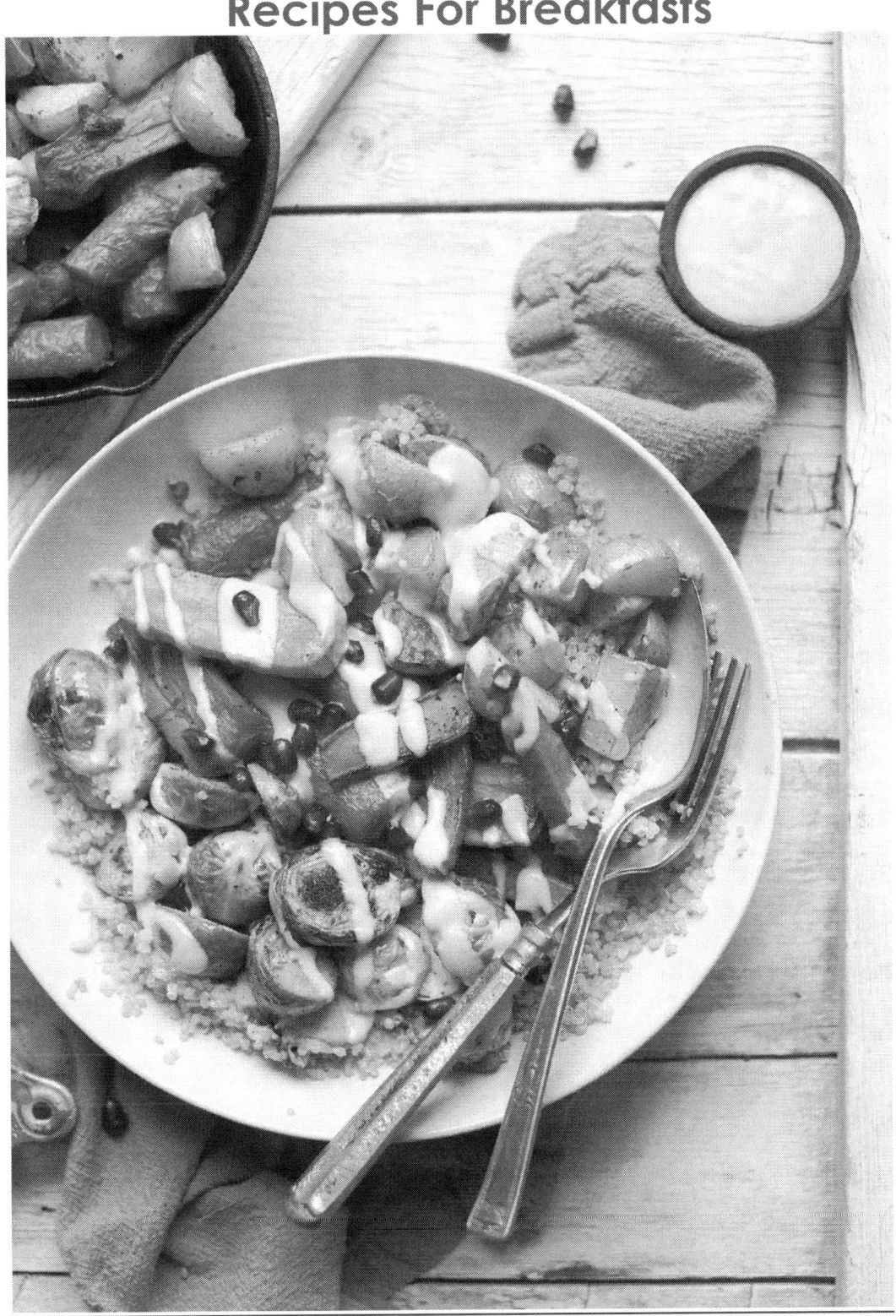

Pancakes – 6 SmartPoints®

Ingredients:

1 tsp. sweetener, artificial
1 beaten egg white
½ Tbsp. cinnamon
½ Tbsp. baking powder
½ c. buttermilk
¾ c. whole wheat flour
1/3 c. unsweetened applesauce

Directions:

1. Combine together the egg, sweetener, cinnamon, baking powder, buttermilk, flour, and applesauce inside a bowl until there are no more lumps. Add in a bit of water to help the consistency if it is too thick.
2. *SPRAY A BIT OF COOKING SPRAY ON THE SKILLET AND LET IT HEAT UP. WHEN THE SKILLET IS READY, ADD A BIT OF THE BATTER TO THE SKILLET AND SPREAD IT OUT A BIT.*
3. Let these pancakes cook for a few minutes to allow the bubbles to start forming.
4. At this time, flip over the pancake and let it cook for an additional minute. Take off the heat when done and then repeat the steps with the rest of the batter until done.

Healthy Morning Cookies – 2 SmartPoints®

Ingredients:

2 egg whites
1/3 c. unsweetened cocoa
1/3 c. chocolate chips, mini
½ c. brown sugar, pressed down
½ c. sugar
1/8 tsp. salt
¼ c. butter, softened
1 c. flour
¼ tsp. baking soda

Directions:

1. Turn on the oven and let it heat up to 350 degrees. Take out a cookie sheet and spray it with some cooking spray.
2. *NOW TAKE OUT A BOWL AND MIX TOGETHER THE BAKING SODA, FLOUR, AND SALT. IN A SECOND BOWL, COMBINE THE BUTTER AND THE BROWN SUGAR AND MIX TOGETHER UNTIL FLUFFY.*
3. Add in the sugar to this second bowl and continue to beat to make it well incorporated. Put all of this into the flour mixture and keep on stirring to combine. Now add in the chocolate chips.
4. Place small amounts of this onto the cookie sheet and then put into the oven and let it bake for about 10 minutes.
5. *TAKE OUT OF THE OVEN AND ALLOW THE COOKIES TO COOL DOWN FOR A FEW MINUTES BEFORE TAKING THEM OFF THE PAN AND COOLING DOWN COMPLETELY.*

Cinnamon Rolls—6 SmartPoints

Ingredients:

¼ c. cream cheese
¼ c. sugar
¼ tsp. vanilla
1 tsp. butter, melted
11 oz. breadstick dough, cold
2 Tbsp. brown sugar
1 tsp. cinnamon

Directions:

1. Turn on the oven and let it heat up to 375 degrees. While that is heating up, take out a baking pan and prepare it with some cooking spray.
2. Take out a small bowl and mix together the brown sugar, cinnamon, and the butter and place to the side.
3. Take the breadstick dough and make it into 12 strips. Sprinkle on some brown sugar to this dough and then roll them into a spiral. Press the dough down to seal up the ends.
4. Place these rolls into a baking pan, leaving them about an inch apart. Place into the oven and let them bake for 15 minutes. When they are done, take out of the oven and let them cool for 10 minutes.
5. While the rolls are baking, work on the frosting. Bring out a bowl and mix together the cream cheese, sugar, and vanilla. Add a bit of water to this until you get the consistency that you would like.
6. Drizzle this frosting onto the prepared rolls and let it set for a few minutes before serving.

Mushroom and Spinach Quiche – 3 SmartPoints®

Ingredients:

Salt
Pepper
¼ c. chopped onion
3 eggs
½ c. cottage cheese
2 tsp. garlic, minced
1 c. artichoke hearts, chopped
½ tsp. olive oil
10 oz. spinach
1 c. mushrooms, sliced

Directions:

1. Turn on the oven and let it heat up to 350 degrees. While that is heating up, take out a pan and cook together the olive oil, mushrooms, onions, and garlic.
2. When those are ready, add in the spinach and let it cook for a bit. After a few minutes, add in the rest of the ingredients and season with some pepper and salt.
3. Place this into a prepared pie dish and let it bake for 45 minutes before serving.

Apple Muffin – 7 SmartPoints®

Ingredients:

½ c. milk
2 Tbsp. vegetable oil
½ tsp. salt
½ tsp. cinnamon
1 ½ tsp. baking powder
1 c. oats
½ tsp. baking soda
2/3 c. brown sugar
2 c. shredded apple
1 ½ c. flour, all purpose

Directions:

1. Turn on the oven and let it heat up to 375 degrees. In the meantime, take out a muffin pan and grease it up.
2. Take out a bowl and combine together the milk, cinnamon, vegetable oil, baking soda, salt, brown sugar, baking powder, flour, and oats.
3. When this is all combined, pour the batter inside the muffin tin and then place into the oven.
4. Allow these to bake for 18 minutes or until they are all done. Give them some time to cool down before serving.

Potato and Cheese Casserole – 7 SmartPoints®

Ingredients:

Salt
Pepper
4 beaten eggs
1 can milk, evaporated
3 oz. bacon, chopped
½ c. scallion, sliced
3 c. potato, shredded
¾ c. cheddar cheese

Directions:

1. For this recipe, turn on the oven and let it heat up to 350 degrees. Take out your baking pan and coat it with some cooking spray.
2. Place the potatoes into the prepared baking pan and then top with some cheese, scallions, and bacon.
3. Now bring out a small bowl and mix together the pepper, salt, eggs, and milk inside. Pour this all on top of the potato mixture.
4. Place this meal inside the oven and let it cook for 40 minutes or until everything has time to set.
5. Take it out of the oven and give it a few minutes to cool down before slicing and enjoying.

Crispy Apple Surprise – 11 SmartPoints®

Ingredients:

Ground cloves
3 lb. sliced apples
¼ c. sugar
1 tsp. vanilla
¼ tsp. nutmeg
3 Tbsp. butter
1 tsp. water
¼ tsp. cinnamon
Salt
¼ c. brown sugar
½ tsp. ginger
½ c. and 2 Tbsp. flour
½ c. quick cooking oats

Directions;

1. For this recipe, turn on the oven and let it heat up to 375 degrees. Take out a baking dish and cover it with some cooking spray.
2. First we will need to make the topping. To do this, bring out a bowl and combine the oats with the cinnamon, salt, brown sugar, ginger, and ½ cup of flour.
3. Add in the butter at this time and then place it all into the pastry blender so that you get a nice crumbly mixture. Pour in some water and then press this to make clumps.
4. Now you will want to work on the filling. To do this, bring out a bowl and combine the cloves, sugar, nutmeg, and the rest of the flour. Put in the vanilla and the apples in as well and then pour everything inside a baking dish.
5. Pour your topping over the filling and then place everything into the oven. Bake this all in the oven for 60 minutes.

Breakfast Jelly Pudding – 11 SmartPoints®

Ingredients:

16 oz. fruit cocktail, canned
16 oz. mandarin orange, canned
1/3 oz. raspberry Jell-O, sugar free
20 oz. pineapple, canned
16 oz. whipped cream
1 oz. vanilla pudding mix

Directions:

1. Take out the canned fruits and take all of the liquid out of them. Bring out a bowl and combine the pudding mix, gelatin, and whipped cream.
2. Slowly fold in the fruits that you just drained out and then chill for a few hours inside the fridge before serving.

Pumpkin Muffins – 4 SmartPoints®

Ingredients:

18 oz. spice cake mix
15 oz. pumpkin
1 c. water

Directions:

1. For this recipe, turn on the oven and let it heat up to 375 degrees.
2. While the oven is heating up, take out a bowl and combine the water, pumpkin, and spice cake mix.
3. Prepare a muffin pan and then pour the batter inside of it. Place these into the oven and bake until it is all done before serving.

Blackberry and Peach Smoothie – 9 SmartPoints®

Ingredients:

½ c. skim milk
¾ c. ice cubes
¼ c. blackberries
2 peeled peaches, sliced

Directions:

1. Bring out a blender and add in the milk, ice cubes, blackberries, and peaches.
2. Turn on the blender and let it process all of the ingredients until they are smooth.
3. Pour this into your favorite cup and then serve!

Morning Burritos – 9 SmartPoints®

Ingredients:
½ c. sour cream
½ c. salsa
¼ tsp. pepper
4 tortillas
2 Tbsp. cilantro
¼ tsp. salt
4 egg whites
½ c. cheddar cheese
2 chopped garlic cloves
2 eggs
1 diced green pepper
½ c. tomato, chopped
2 tsp. olive oil
1/3 c. scallions, chopped
Directions:

1. To start this recipe, turn on the oven and let it heat up to 400 degrees. Take out a baking pan and spray it with some cooking spray.
2. Now you can add in a bit of oil to the skillet and add in the tomato garlic, scallions, and green pepper. Let this cook for about 5 minutes.

3. After this time, add in the eggs and the egg whites and cook for another five minutes. Take everything off the heat at this time.
4. Add in the salt, pepper, cheese, and cilantro.
5. Lay out the tortillas and scoop a bit of the filling into each one. Roll them up tight and then place into the baking pan.
6. Bake these in the oven for 10 minutes. Serve with a bit of salsa and some sour cream and then enjoy!

Breakfast Souffle – 3 SmartPoints®

Ingredients:
1/8 tsp. cayenne pepper
2 eggs
2 egg whites
1 ½ c. cheddar cheese
½ tsp. salt
3 Tbsp. flour
1 c. milk
Directions:

1. Take out a bowl and mix three tablespoons of the milk together with the flour and set to the side.
2. Place the rest of the milk into a pan and let it cook over a low heat. Add the flour mixture to this pan and then cook it while stirring the whole time so that it can begin to thicken.
3. Remove this from the heat and then put in a bit of salt and the cayenne pepper and cheese. Move this over to a bowl and let it cool down.
4. Turn on the oven on to 350 degrees. While that is heating up, add the egg yolks into the cheese mixture until they are well incorporated.
5. Bring out a glass bowl and whip up all the egg whites together. Combine ¼ of these with the cheese mixture and then fold in the rest of the beaten egg with our rubber spatula.
6. Place this mixture into a soufflé dish and then bake in the oven for about 35 minutes. Serve right away when it is done.

Breakfast Bars – 6 SmartPoints®

Ingredients:

1 tsp. vanilla
1/3 c. water
¾ c. chocolate chips
6 Tbsp. butter
2 egg whites
½ tsp. salt
2 c. flour
2 tsp. baking powder

Directions:

1. Turn on the oven and let it heat up to 350 degrees. While that is heating up, bring out a bowl and mix together the salt, baking powder, and flour.
2. In another bowl, mix together the butter and the brown sugar until they are nice and fluffy before adding in the egg whites and the vanilla. Slowly whisk in the flour mixture and alternate it with a bit of water as well.
3. Add in the chocolate chips and mix them in well. Place some foil onto a baking pan and then pour the mixture on the pan.
4. Place this into the oven and let it bake for 25 minutes. Let the bars cool on a wire rack when you are done. Cut into slices when you are ready and enjoy.

French Toast – 3 SmartPoints®

Ingredients:
6 slices wheat bread
1 pkg. sugar free maple syrup
1 Tbsp. cinnamon
1 Tbsp. vanilla
Cooking spray
4 egg whites
¼ c. skim milk

Directions:

1. To start this recipe, bring out a bowl and mix together the egg whites and the vanilla.

2. Take out a skillet and grease it u with some cooking spray. Heat up the skillet.
3. While the skillet is heating up, dip the bread slices in the egg mixture and let each side get nice and soaked. Allow the extra batter to drip off.
4. Place the bread onto the skillet and let each side cook for about 3 minutes. Place these onto a plate and serve.

Cheese and Ham Omelet – 6 SmartPoints®

Ingredients:

½ c. diced ham
¼ c. Parmesan cheese
1/8 tsp. pepper
1/8 tsp. hot pepper sauce
2 Tbsp. green onion, chopped
¼ tsp. salt
2 eggs
4 egg whites

Directions:

1. For this recipe, bring out a bowl and ix together the hot sauce, salt, pepper, eggs, and onion.
2. Take out a skillet and grease it with some cooking spray before heating it up. Pour the mixture into the skillet and let it cook for 5 minutes so it has time to set.
3. Sprinkle the top with the ham and the Parmesan cheese. Fold the omelet in half and let it cook for another minute before serving.

Spiced Honey Cake – 7 SmartPoints®

Ingredients:
1 tsp. grated orange zest
2 Tbsp. canola oil
½ c. honey
¼ c. sliced almonds
2 eggs
¼ c. white sugar
½ tsp. nutmeg
½ tsp. cloves
1 tsp. cinnamon
¾ tsp. allspice
½ tsp. baking soda
1/8 tsp. salt
1 ½ c. flour
¾ tsp. baking powder
½ c. applesauce

Directions:

1. To start this recipe, turn on the oven and let it heat up to 350 degrees. Grease up a loaf pan using some cooking spray and set it to the side.
2. Mix together the nutmeg, cloves, cinnamon, allspice, baking soda, salt, four, and baking powder. When this is combined, set it aside.
3. In another bowl, beat together the eggs until they are frothy. Add in the sugar, honey, and oil and mix to make this a pale yellow before adding in the orange zest and apple sauce.
4. Slowly combined in the wet mixture and the dry mixture, making sure to combine them together well. When these are read, pour inside a loaf pan and then top with some almonds.
5. Place all of this into the oven and let it bake for about 40 minutes until it is cooked all the way through.
6. Allow the cake to cool down for another 20 minutes before serving.

Blueberry Muffins – 5 SmartPoints®

Ingredients:
2 ½ c. hot water
1 ½ tsp. baking powder
3 c. bran cereal
19 oz. blueberry muffin mix
Directions:

1. Turn on the oven and let it heat up to 400 degrees. Prepare a muffin pan using some paper liners or with some cooking spray.
2. While the oven is heating up, combine the hot water and the bran cereal together and then set them to the side.
3. Bring out another bowl so that you can mix together the baking powder and the muffin mix. When these are combined, place the bran cereal and water so that they can be incorporated as well.
4. Pour this batter inside of your prepared muffin pan and then bake for 15 minutes or until the muffins are cooked all the way through.

Yogurt Fluff – 2 SmartPoints®

Ingredients:

12 tsp. vanilla
Ice cubes
½ c. cold water
1 c. yogurt
¾ c. boiling water
8 ½ grams cherry gelatin

Directions:

1. Combine together the gelatin and the boiling water inside of a bowl and ix so that the gelatin is completely dissolved.
2. Put the ice cubes into some cold water and then get a cup of this mixture. Pour this into the gelatin and continue to mix so that it can become thicker. Get rid of any ice that is extra.

3. Add in the yogurt as well as the vanilla and let it stir until it becomes well blended.
4. Place the bowl into the fridge and let it chill for at least 30 minutes. After this time add in some whipped cream and enjoy!

Recipes For Lunches

Living Sweet Moments

Creamy Pesto Pasta – 7 SmartPoints®

Ingredients:

1 tsp. lemon juice
1 ½ tsp. olive oil
2 ½ Tbsp. cream cheese
2 garlic cloves
4 ½ c. baby spinach
2 Tbsp. water
1 ¼ tsp. salt
8 oz. uncooked spaghetti

Directions:

1. For this recipe, take out a pot of water and boil it with a bit of salt. Add in the pasta and let it cook for 8 minutes or until it is all done.
2. Drain out the water and top with some cherry tomatoes and Parmesan cheese. Process the salt, oil, garlic, spinach, and water inside the blender until it is soft.
3. Add in the cream cheese to the pasta until it melts. Then add in the reserved pasta water and the pesto sauce and mix to get the right consistency.
4. Season with some lemon juice and salt and then enjoy.

BBQ Pork Sandwich – 5 SmartPoints®

Ingredients:

1 cut bell pepper, green
6 hamburger buns
12 oz. pork tenderloin
¼ tsp. salt
1 tsp. Worcestershire sauce
1 Tbsp. brown sugar
1 ½ tsp. chili powder
6 oz. can tomato paste
2 Tbsp. red wine vinegar
2 minced garlic cloves
2/3 c. water
1 minced onion

Directions:

1. Grease up a small pan with some cooking spray and then heat it up. Add in the onion and the garlic and let these cook for 5 minutes.
2. At this time, add in the oregano, Worcestershire sauce, brown sugar, chili powder, tomato paste, vinegar, and garlic. Bring all of this to a boil.
3. Simmer this without the top on for about 10 minutes so that the liquid can reduce a bit, making sure to stir occasionally.
4. While that is cooking, take the meat and remove the fat a bit. Cut this meat into smaller strips. Take out another skillet and brush with some cooking spray.
5. Season the meat with some salt and place the meat in the skillet. Cook the meat for three minutes before pouring in the bell peppers and sauce.
6. Cook all of the ingredients together for a few minutes. When it is ready, serve the pork on toasted buns and enjoy.

Italian Chicken – 5 SmartPoints®

Ingredients:

Juice from two lemons
Pepper
Salt
2 Tbsp. capers
¼ c. parsley, chopped
½ c. chicken broth
2 Tbsp. butter
1 ½ lbs. chicken breast, sliced
¾ c. white wine

Directions:

1. To start up this recipe, turn on the oven and let it heat up to 350 degrees. Lay out the chicken breasts onto a board and then cover with some cling wrap. Flatten the chicken with a mallet to make them ¼ inch thick.
2. Season the chicken with the pepper and salt and then move this over to a baking dish. Add some butter to the chicken and then surround it with the broth, wine, and lemon juice.
3. Sprinkle everything with the capers and then cover with some foil before placing into the oven and baking for 20 minutes.
4. Remove the foil after this time and then bake them for an additional 10 minutes. Sprinkle with some parsley and then serve right away.

Baked Tortellini – 6 SmartPoints®

Ingredients:
2/3 c. mozzarella cheese
2 tsp. lemon zest
2 c. spinach
¼ tsp. red pepper flakes
1 Tbsp. lemon juice
1/8 tsp. pepper
1 ½ tsp. basil
¾ tsp. salt
2 Tbsp. flour
2 c. milk
2 bacon slices
3 chopped garlic cloves
12 oz. dry spinach and cheese
1 pkg. tortellini
1 ½ oz. Parmesan cheese
Directions:

1. Turn on the oven and let it heat up to 350 degrees. While that is heating up, take out a baking dish and cover with some cooking spray.
2. Follow the directions on the package and cook the tortellini. In the meantime, place the bacon into a skillet and cook for 9 minutes so it becomes crisp. Take the bacon off the skillet and put on a paper towel to absorb the oil. Save some of this bacon grease.
3. Add the garlic into the bacon grease and let it cook for a minute before adding in the flour and whisk in the milk. Now add in the basil, red pepper flakes, and pepper.
4. Bring all of this to a simmer and then add in the lemon juice and lemon zest and let t stir for another 3 minutes.
5. Take all of this off the heat. Crumble up the bacon and set it to the side. Mix the mozzarella, spinach, parmesan, and tortellini together.
6. Move this mixture to the baking dish and top with the rest of the bacon, Parmesan, and mozzarella.
7. Cover this with foil and place into the oven to bake for 20 minutes. Remove the foil at this time and then bake for another 10 minutes before serving.

Cheesy Mushrooms – 2 SmartPoints®

Ingredients:

½ tsp. olive oil
1/8 tsp. cayenne pepper
1 tsp. lemon juice
½ tsp. lemon zest
2 Tbsp. feta cheese
½ Tbsp. parsley
8 mushrooms
2 pieces mushroom stems

Directions:

1. Turn on the oven and let it heat up to 425 degrees. Bring out a baking dish and let it get covered with cooking spray.
2. Rinse the mushrooms and dry them with some paper towels. Pull the stems off the mushrooms and set two of these to the side. Mince up the mushroom stems and place into a bowl.
3. Place the mushrooms into the baking dish and then mx in the rest of the ingredients with the minced stems. Place this mixture into the caps of the mushrooms.
4. Place this into the oven and let it bake for about 15 minutes. Allow this some time to cool down before serving.

Baked Burrito – 6 SmartPoints®

Ingredients:

¼ c. water
1 c. Mexican cheese
10 oz. canned refried beans
1 c. Bisquick
1 c. mozzarella cheese
1 lb. ground beef
1 pack taco seasoning

Directions:

1. Cook up the ground beef and until it is cooked all the way through and then drain out the liquid. Add in the taco seasoning and let it simmer.
2. Bring out another bowl and combine the refried beans with the Bisquick and water. Put this mixture into a pan and then top with some cheese and beef.
3. Turn on the oven to 350 degrees and then add in the meal. Bake this for 30 minutes and then serve.

Italian Bread with some Tuna Salad – 10 SmartPoints®

Ingredients:

8 oz. Italian bread
2 tomatoes, sliced
¼ tsp. salt
1 tsp. dried oregano
½ tsp. pepper
3 Tbsp. balsamic vinegar
1 red onion, sliced
1 Tbsp. capers, rinsed or drained.
4 c. lettuce, shredded
8 oz. white tuna

Directions:

1. Start by making the tuna salad part. Mix together the onion, capers, lettuce, and tuna. Set this to the side.

2. Then you can go on and make the dressing. To do this, you will be able to mix together the salt, pepper, garlic, oregano, vinegar, olive oil. Drizzle this on top of the tuna salad and toss around to combine.
3. Next it is time to make the sandwiches. You can cut the bread lengthwise and then spread it open. Arrange the tomatoes on the bottom of the bread.
4. Top this all with the salad mixture and then wrap up the sandwich with some cling wrap. Chill in the fridge for a few hours before serving.

Turkey and Cheese Sandwich – 10 SmartPoints®

Ingredients:

8 slices of bread
4 oz. sliced cheese
½ c. milk
4 tsp. Dijon mustard
4 oz. sliced chicken breast
1 egg
1 egg white

Directions:

1. Take out a small bowl and whisk together the milk, egg, and egg white. Lay out the bread and layer with some of the mustard on top.
2. Top the bread slices with some turkey and cheese. Put the rest of the bread slices on top of them to put the sandwiches together.
3. Grease a pan with some cooking spray and then place over the heat. Coat each of the sandwiches with the egg mixture and place inside a hot pan.
4. Cook the sandwiches for about 4 minutes on each side before serving.

Veggie Soup – 1 SmartPoint

Ingredients:

1 tsp. Cajun spices
¼ tsp. basil
2 beef bouillon cubs
½ c. zucchini slices
2 minced garlic cloves
14 ½ oz. canned tomatoes, diced
2 ½ c. cabbage, shredded
1 ½ stalks chopped celery
14 oz. canned beef broth
½ sliced onion
1 c. sliced carrot

Directions:

1. Spray a pan with some cooking spray and then add inn the celery, onions, and carrots inside.
2. Take out a big pot and mx together the basil, garlic, Cajun spice, cabbage, bouillon cubes, beef broth, and tomatoes together. Add in the vegetables you just cooked as well.
3. Bring all of this to a boil and let it simmer together for about 30 minutes.
4. After this time, put the zucchini into the pot and simmer for an additional 10 minutes. Serve it warm.

Cheeseburger Soup – 7 SmartPoints®

Ingredients:
1/8 tsp. pepper
24 pieces corn tortilla chips
½ tsp. paprika
¼ tsp. salt
1 c. evaporated milk
8 oz. cubed Velveeta
2 Tbsp. flour
3 c. chicken broth
1 chopped celery stalk
1 lb. uncooked ground beef
1 chopped garlic clove
1 diced onion
Cooking spray

Directions:

1. Take out a skillet and spray on some cooking spray. Add on the celery, garlic, and onion and let these cook until they are tender.

2. Bring out a slow cooker and spray with some cooking spray. Transfer these over to the slow cooker.

3. Take out another skillet and cook the beef for about six minutes or until it is cooked through. Move this over to the slow cooker.

4. In another bowl, mix together ½ cup of the broth so that you can get rid of the lumps. Put the flour into the skillet and add in the rest 2 ½ cups of broth inside.

5. Let this simmer, taking time to take the browned bits off the bottom of the skillet. When this is done, move it over to the slow cooker and add in the pepper, paprika, salt, evaporated milk, and cheese.

6. Place the lid into the slow cooker and let it cook on a low setting for 2 hours. Pour your flour mixture inside the slow cooker at this time.

7. Cover the slow cooker and let this cook for another 15 minutes. When you are ready to serve, add some crushed tortilla chips and enjoy.

Pasta Veggies – 5 SmartPoints®

Ingredients:

½ c. mayo
2 Tbsp. scallions, sliced
½ tsp. red pepper
¼ c. celery, diced
¾ c. salsa
½ yellow bell pepper
½ c. cherry tomatoes
6 oz. pasta
12 oz. tuna, canned

Directions:

1. Cook the pasta by following the directions on the package. When this is done, drain out the pasta and rinse it under some cold water. Then drain it again.
2. Now you can bring out a big bowl and mix together the celery, bell pepper, tomatoes, pasta, and tuna.
3. In a second bowl, combine the red pepper, salsa, and mayo together. Pour this dressing over the pasta mixture and toss it together well.
4. Cover the bowl and then place into the fridge to chill for a bit. Right before serving, top with some scallions and enjoy.

Bacon Wrap – 8 SmartPoints®

Ingredients:

½ lb. sliced roast beef
2 sliced tomatoes
¼ tsp. pepper
7 pieces tortilla
2 tsp. Dijon mustard
2 c. shredded lettuce
¼ tsp. salt
1/3 c. basil
1/3 c. mayo

Directions:

1. Bring out a bowl and combine the pepper, Dijon mustard, salt, basil, and mayo.
2. Lay out the tortillas and spread the mixture from above all over it.
3. Sprinkle the tortillas with some lettuce, roast beef, and tomatoes. Roll this up and then serve.

Baked Fish – 5 SmartPoints®

Ingredients:

½ tsp. paprika
1/3 c. milk
½ tsp. salt
3 Tbsp. melted butter
1/8 tsp. pepper
¼ c. bread crumbs
½ tsp. dill
1 ½ lb. white fish fillet
¼ c. yellow cornmeal

Directions:

1. Turn on the oven and let it heat up to 450 degrees. Bring out a pie plate and combine together all of your dry ingredients.

2. Add in the milk to another milk. Dip the fish inside the milk to coat and then put it through the crumb mixture.
3. Place the fish into a greased pan and then drizzle the fish with some melted butter.
4. Bake the fish for 10 minutes and then serve with your favorite sides.

Beef Ziti Bake – 7 SmartPoints®

Ingredients:

20 oz. crushed tomatoes
1 c. mozzarella cheese
1 tsp. oregano
1 tsp. thyme
¼ tsp. pepper
1/3 lb. ground beef
½ tsp. salt
2 minced garlic cloves
12 oz. ziti
2 tsp. olive oil

Directions:

1. Turn on the oven and let it heat up to 350 degrees. Cook the ziti by following the directions on the package. When this is done, drain out the pasta and rinse it off.
2. Heat up some olive oil into a pan and then cook the garlic inside for a minute. Cook the ground beef in here, seasoning with some pepper and salt, and cook all the way through.
3. Remove the fat and then mix in the thyme, rosemary, and oregano and cook for two more minutes. Add in the tomatoes and bring to a boil to simmer for five minutes.
4. Bring out a casserole dish and put some of the meat sauce to cover all of the bottom. Put in half of your prepared ziti and then the rest of the meat sauce. Now add in half of the mozzarella cheese and then finish the layers.
5. Bake the ziti in the oven for 30 minutes so the cheese has time to melt the cheese before serving.

Chicken Salad – 4 SmartPoints®

Ingredients:

½ tsp. salt
¼ tsp. pepper
1 tsp. Dijon mustard
1 tsp. lemon juice
2 Tbsp. sour cream
2 Tbsp. parsley
1/3 c. dill pickle
¼ c. mayo
1 lb. chicken breast
½ c. celery, chopped

Directions:

1. Take out a pan and place the chicken inside. Add in just enough water to cover up the chicken. Bring this all to a boil.
2. Allow the chicken to boil for 10 minutes and then drain out the liquid, allowing the chicken to cool a bit.
3. Slice the chicken into small cubes and then place the chicken into a bowl.
4. *At this time, add in the pepper, salt, lemon juice, parsley, mustard, mayo, sour cream, celery, and pickles together. Toss around to coat and serve.*

Egg Salad – 4 SmartPoints®

Ingredients:
¼ tsp. pepper
½ tsp. salt
1 piece of dill
2 Tbsp. mayo
½ tsp. Dijon mustard
2 Tbsp. chives
4 eggs
2 hard boiled eggs

Directions:

1. Bring out a pan and fill it with the water and the eggs. Place this on a high heat and bring it to a boil.

2. When the eggs are done, drain the water out and add in the eggs to an ice water bath. When the eggs are cooled down, you can remove the shells from the eggs.
3. Also take some time to remove the yolks from two the eggs. Slice up the eggs into smaller pieces and add into a bowl.
4. Add in the pepper, salt, mustard, dill, chives, and mayo to the bowl and stir well before serving.

Beef Burgers – 4 SmartPoints®

Ingredients;

½ tsp. salt
¼ tsp. pepper
Four hamburger buns, low calorie
1 Tbsp. Worcestershire sauce
2 tsp. garlic, minced
Cooking spray
1 lb. ground beef
Directions:

1. Coat your griddle with some cooking spray and heat it up. Take out a bowl and add in the pepper, salt, Worcestershire sauce, garlic, and beef. Form this into patties.
2. Place the burgers onto the prepared griddle and cook the patties for five minutes on each side.
3. Add some of our favorite toppings and then enjoy.

Recipes For Dinners

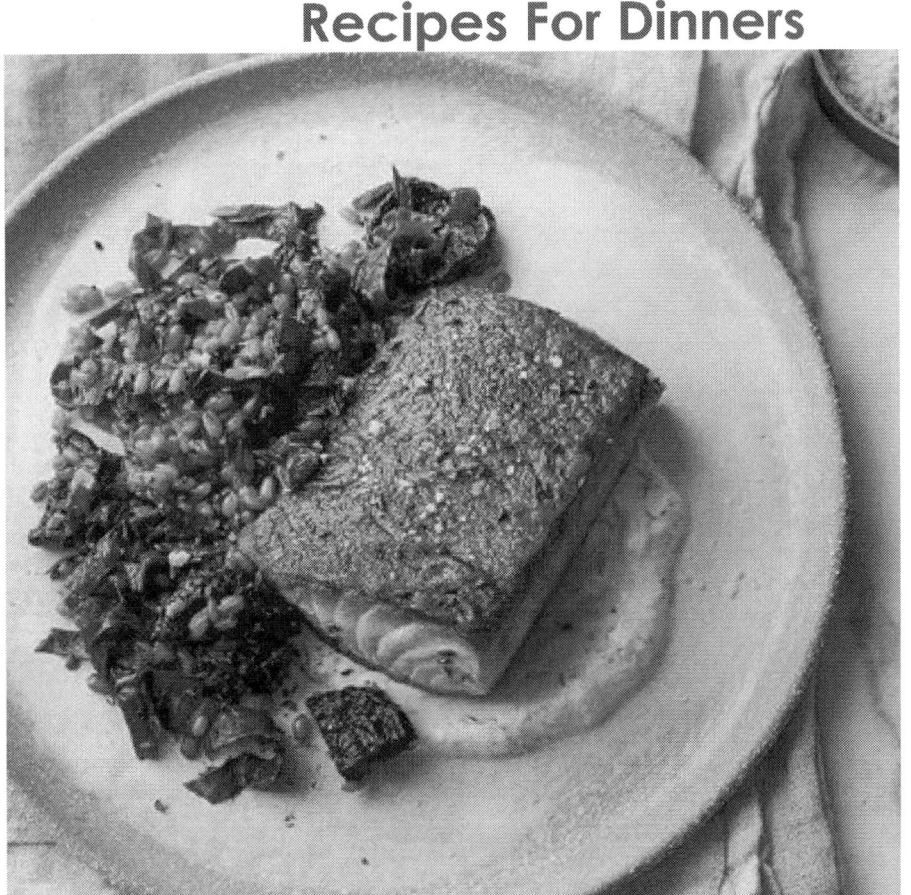

Cheesy Chicken Chops -3 Smart Points

Ingredients:
½ tsp. garlic powder
¼ tsp. pepper
1 lb. chicken breast
1/8 tsp. paprika
1 tsp. parsley
¼ c. parmesan cheese
2 Tbsp. dried Italian bread crumbs
Directions:
1.   Turn on the oven and let it heat up to 400 degrees. Bring out a bag and add in the seasonings, cheese, and crumbs and mix them together.
2.   Move this mixture over to a plate. Coat the chicken in this cheese mixture and then move over to a baking sheet.

3.   Allow this to bake inside the air fryer for about 25 minutes or until it is cooked through and then serve.

Jalapeno Chicken – 5 SmartPoints®

Ingredients:
2 Tbsp. Worcestershire sauce
16 oz. chicken breasts
1 tsp. garlic powder
1/3 c. steak sauce
1/3 c. jalapeno jelly, melted
Directions:
1.   Bring out a small bowl and mix together the Worcestershire sauce, garlic powder, steak sauce, and jalapeno jelly.
2.   Add the chicken into this mixture and let it marinate inside the fridge overnight.
3.   Spray the griddle with some cooking spray. Cook the chicken for about 5 minutes on each side so that the chicken can cook through.

Cilantro Lime Shrimp – 3 SmartPoints®

Ingredients:
¼ tsp. pepper
¼ c. cilantro, chopped
1 tsp. lime zest, grated
2 minced garlic cloves
1 Tbsp. olive oil
½ tsp. cumin
¼ tsp. ginger
1 ¾ lb. shrimp
2 Tbsp. lime juice
½ tsp. salt
Directions;
1.   To make this simple recipe, bring out a bowl and mix together the garlic, cumin, ginger, shrimp, and lime juice.
2.   Heat up some oil inside a skillet and then add in the shrimp. Let it cook inside the skillet for about 4 minutes.
3.   Before serving, garnish with some pepper, salt, cilantro, and lime zest.

Spinach and Chicken Crescents -4 SmartPoints®

Ingredients:
1 c. baby spinach
1/3 c. Mexican blend cheese
5 oz. chicken strips, grilled
8 oz. crescent roll dough
4 Tbsp. cream cheese, soft

Directions:

1.   Turn on the oven and let it heat up to 375 degrees. Put the crescent rolls onto a baking sheet and put some spinach and cream cheese on top of the rolls.

2.   Grill up the chicken strips if you need to and then place these on the crescent with the Mexican cheese.

3.   Tuck in the roll to wrap up the filling and then bake the meal for about 14 minutes inside the oven before serving.

Steak and Mashed Potatoes – 8 SmartPoints®

Ingredients;

1 ½ c. beef broth
4 cube steaks
Pepper
8 oz. sliced mushrooms
4 Tbsp. flour
1 lb. diced potatoes
½ tsp. salt

Directions:

1.   To start this recipe, bring out a pot and boil and simmer the potatoes until they are nice and tender. Drain these out when you are done and keep ½ cup of the liquid.

2.   Season the cooked potatoes with some pepper and salt and then mash them up using the liquid that you reserved.

3.   Mix together some of the extra liquid with 2 tablespoon flour. Cover the steaks with the remaining flour as well as some salt and pepper and then cook the steaks for about 2 minutes on each side.

4.   Mix in the mushrooms to this mixture and bring it all to a boil. When it reaches a boil, simmer the ingredients for 30 minutes.

5.   Remove the cover at this time and cook so the gravy can thicken. Serve with some of the mashed potatoes and enjoy.

Honey Salmon – 4 SmartPoints®

Ingredients:
½ tsp. pepper
¼ c. sliced scallions
1 lb. salmon fillets
½ tsp. salt
1 tsp. ginger
2 tsp. wasabi
1 Tbsp. soy sauce
1 Tbsp. honey
3 Tbsp. mirin
1 Tbsp. rice vinegar
Direction:
1.   **Boil the wasabi, ginger, soy sauce, honey, mirin, and vinegar together in a pan for about five minutes.**
2.   **After this time, take it off the heat and sprinkle with some salt and pepper. Sprinkle with a bit of salt and pepper.**
3.   **Grease up a skillet and let it heat up a little bit. Cook the salmon in the skillet on 4 minutes on both sides.**
4.   **Spoon a bit of the sauce on top of the salmon and then top a bit of the scallions on top of it before serving.**

Veggie Pork Chops – 6 SmartPoints®

Ingredients:
1 ½ tsp. oregano
½ tsp. cumin
2 c. corn
½ c. salsa
1 diced onion
14.5 oz. can stewed tomatoes
16 oz. pork chops
1 diced green peppers
Directions:
1. Turn the oven on and let it heat up to 350 degrees. Cook up the pork chops in a preheated skillet and let it cook for two minutes on each side of the meat.
2. Move the pork over to a prepared casserole dish. Grease up the skillet with some more cooking spray and then add in the rest of the ingredients. Cook these for about five minutes.

3. When these ingredients are well combined, pour this mixture all over the pork chops and then cover the dish with some foil.
4. Bake the pork chops in the oven for about 50 minutes or until the pork is cooked through before serving.

Mexican Casserole – 8 SmartPoints®

Ingredients:

1/3 c. Mexican cheese blend
1/3 chopped cilantro bunch
8 pieces corn tortilla
¾ c. sour cream
15 oz. corn kernels
15 oz. can black beans
¼ c. jalapeno pepper, chopped
2 c. tomato, chopped
1 lb. ground beef
½ c. diced onion

Directions:

1. Bring out our skillet and cook the onions and beef inside for about 12 minutes. Drain and rinse off the meat with some warm water in order to remove some of the fat.
2. Place the meat into the skillet again and add in the taco seasoning mix, tomatoes, jalapenos, corn, and black beans and let this heat and simmer for another five minutes.
3. Cut the 8 tortillas in half and then arrange 8 of the halves into a prepared baking dish. Put half of the beef mixture and the sour cream over the tortillas.
4. Cover with the rest of the tortillas and then the rest of the beef mixture. Turn the oven on to 350 degrees at this time.
5. Bake the dish for about 25 minutes. When this is all done, top with some cilantro and cheese before serving.

Chicken Thai Wrap – 2 SmartPoints®

Ingredients:
½ tsp. grated ginger
1 handful sliced green onions
½ tsp. soy sauce
Hot sauce
1/3 c. cabbage
¼ c. snap peas
1/3 c. red bell pepper strips
2 Tbsp. PB2
1 wheat wrap
2 oz. chicken breast
Directions:

1. Start this recipe by bringing out a bowl and mixing together the green onions and the PB2.
2. Then take out a plate and heat up the tortillas inside of the microwave for about 20 seconds.
3. Place the dressing on top of the tortilla and then add in the vegetables and chicken. Wrap up the tortilla and then enjoy.

Pita Bread Pizza – 9 SmartPoints®

Ingredients:
2 tsp. Parmesan cheese
Pinch of pizza seasoning
10 chopped black olives
½ c. mozzarella cheese
¼ c. mushrooms, sliced
¼ c. green pepper
1 pita bread
¼ c. pizza sauce
Directions:

1. Lay out the pita bread and put the pizza sauce all over it. Top this with the seasoning, mozzarella, parmesan cheese, and vegetables.
2. Spray this with a bit of cooking spray and then place it on a baking pan. Turn on the oven to broil.
3. Put the pita into the oven and let it broil in the oven for 2 minutes to let the cheese melt. Take it out of the oven and let it cool down for a bit before serving.

Potato Soup – 4 SmartPoints®

Ingredients:
1 c. water
6 Tbsp. bacon bits
1 pack of gravy
1 c. skim milk
32 oz. hash browns, non-fat
3 cans chicken broth
Directions:

1. Bring out a pot and coat it with some cooking spray. Heat it up and then add in the hash browns.
2. After a few minutes, add in the chicken broth and bring this to a boil before lowering the heat and letting this come to a simmer.
3. While the hash browns are heating up, take out another bowl and mix together the gravy mix, water, and milk.
4. Pour this mixture in with the cooked potatoes and then add in the bacon bits. Cook this for a little bit longer to allow it time to thicken. Season with some salt and then serve.

Roast Beef with Veggies – 8 SmartPoints®

Ingredients:
14 oz. diced tomatoes
1 pack onion soup mix
4 carrots, chunked
1 onion, quartered
2 roast beef
2 lbs. wedged potatoes
Directions:

1. Place the roast into your slow cooker and then top it with the onion soup mix.
2. When that is organized, add in the carrots, onion, and potatoes and then top with the tomatoes.
3. Place the cover onto the slow cooker and let this cook on a low setting for about 7 hours.

Mushroom Steak – 5 SmartPoints®

Ingredients:

2 tsp. Worcestershire sauce
Parsley
2 Tbsp. flour
2 Tbsp. tomato paste
1/8 tsp. pepper
8 oz. sliced mushrooms
2 c. beef broth
¼ tsp. salt
1 egg
1 egg white
1 lb. ground turkey
½ c. bread crumbs
1 ½ tsp. cooking oil
¾ c. onions, minced
½ tsp. mustard powder
¼ c. water
1 tsp. red wine vinegar

Directions:

1. Take out a skillet and cook the oil and the onions together for about 5 minutes.
2. Bring out a bowl and mix together the black pepper, salt, egg, egg white, ground turkey, bread crumbs, half of the cooked onions, ¼ cup of the beef broth, and the ground beef.
3. When this is all combined, use our hands to form these into 8 patties. Add into the skillet and cook on each side to brown.
4. Add the pepper, salt, and mushrooms into the skillet and cook for another 3 minutes. Then add the patties back inside.
5. While that is cooking, mix together the broth and the flour. Then add in the Worcestershire sauce, mustard powder, vinegar, water, tomato paste, and the rest of the onions.
6. Pour this sauce over the meat and mushrooms in the skillet. Serve it warm.

Cheese and Tuna Sandwich – 10 SmartPoints®

Ingredients:
1 sliced tomato
½ c. cheddar cheese
1 ½ Tbsp. butter
2 Tbsp. spicy brown mustard
1 ½ Tbsp. pickle relish
4 slices bread
5 oz. can tuna
1 ½ Tbsp. mayo
Directions:

1. Bring out a bowl and combine together the pickle relish, drained tuna, and the mayo.
2. Lay out the bread and spread out some butter on one of the slices and then mustard on the other.
3. Put the cheese, tomato, and tuna on the side with the mustard and then place the other two slices on top to make our sandwich.
4. Place these both into a pan and then cover and cook for 3 minutes on both sides. Cut in half and then enjoy!

Cola Chicken – 5 SmartPoints®

Ingredients:
1 can of diet cola
½ c. onion, chopped
4 chicken breasts, skinless
1 c. ketchup
Directions:

1. Bring out a skillet to start this recipe and combine the cola and the ketchup inside.
2. After a few minutes, add in the chicken and the onions and stir it all around. Bring this to a boil before placing the cover on top and reducing the heat.
3. Simmer the whole meal together for about 45 minutes so that the chicken has time to marinate before serving.

Tender Beef Chili – 4 SmartPoints®

Ingredients:

2 Tbsp. tomato paste
Pepper
1 chopped sweet onion
¼ c. diced green chilies
28 oz. tomatoes in a can
15 oz. red kidney beans,
2 Tbsp. chili powder
2 tsp. cumin
1 diced red bell pepper
1 diced green bell pepper
1 lb. ground turkey or beef
1 Tbsp. minced garlic

Directions:

1. To start this recipe, bring out a skillet and brown the ground beef together with the garlic. When these are done cooking, take the fat out of the skillet and then add in the bell peppers.
2. Cook this for 5 minutes so that the peppers can get nice and soft. Now add in the chili powder and cumin and cook for a few more minutes.
3. Bring out a slow cooker and add in the meat mixture, tomato paste, chilies, onion, tomatoes, and kidney beans inside.
4. Put the lid on top of the slow cooker and let this cook for about 5 hours. When you are ready to serve, season with some black pepper and serve.

Vegetable Quesadilla – 9 SmartPoints®

Ingredients:

Cooking spray
¼ c. shredded cheddar cheese
¼ c. shredded mozzarella cheese
Salt
2 wheat flour tortillas
1 dash cayenne pepper
Pepper
1 Tbsp. red bell pepper, diced
1 tsp. soy sauce
1/3 c. shredded carrot
1/3 c. broccoli, chopped
½ Tbsp. canola oil
½ c. mushrooms, sliced

Directions:

1. To start this recipe, bring out a pan and cook up the vegetables inside for 7 minutes to make it nice and soft. Season with the salt, soy sauce, and the peppers.
2. When the vegetables are all done cooking place them into the bowl.
3. Clean out the pan if needed and place one of the tortillas inside. Top with half the cheese, some vegetables, and then the remainder of the cheese. Place the second tortilla on top.
4. Heat this for about 2 minutes to make it nice and warm. After that time, turn the quesadilla over and let it cook for another minute before serving.

Baked Chicken – 10 SmartPoints®

Ingredients:

2 Tbsp. Worcestershire sauce
2 tsp. dry mustard
3 Tbsp. brown sugar
2 Tbsp. vinegar
4 chicken breasts
½ c. ketchup

Directions:

1. Turn on the oven and let it heat up to 350 degrees.
2. While the oven is heating up, place the chicken into the baking dish and then add in the ketchup, vinegar, brown sugar, dry mustard, and Worcestershire sauce all around the chicken.
3. Place these into the oven and bake the meal for 40 minutes. Allow some time to cool down before serving.

Chicken and Dumplings – 9 SmartPoints®

Ingredients:
Tortillas
Pepper
Salt
½ Tbsp. celery salt
3 c. chicken breast, chopped
2 cans chicken broth
1 can cream of chicken soup

Directions:
1. Take out a pan and add together the chicken breast, cream of chicken soup, and chicken broth. Sprinkle in the seasonings.
2. Add the tortillas one at a time. Reduce the heat and let it simmer for 25 minutes.

WEIGHT WATCHERS FREESTYLE
SHOPPING LIST

Dry Food:

_____
_____
_____
_____
_____
_____

Fresh Dry Food:

_____
_____
_____
_____
_____

Frozen Food:

_____
_____
_____
_____
_____
_____

Cooking Spices:

_____
_____
_____
_____
_____

Baked Goods:

_____
_____
_____
_____
_____

Miscellaneous

_____
_____
_____
_____
_____

In the next section, I've included my favorite recipes that I could recommend, Although, points is of the old smart points system but never the less still usable and as tasty as always, so let enjoy!

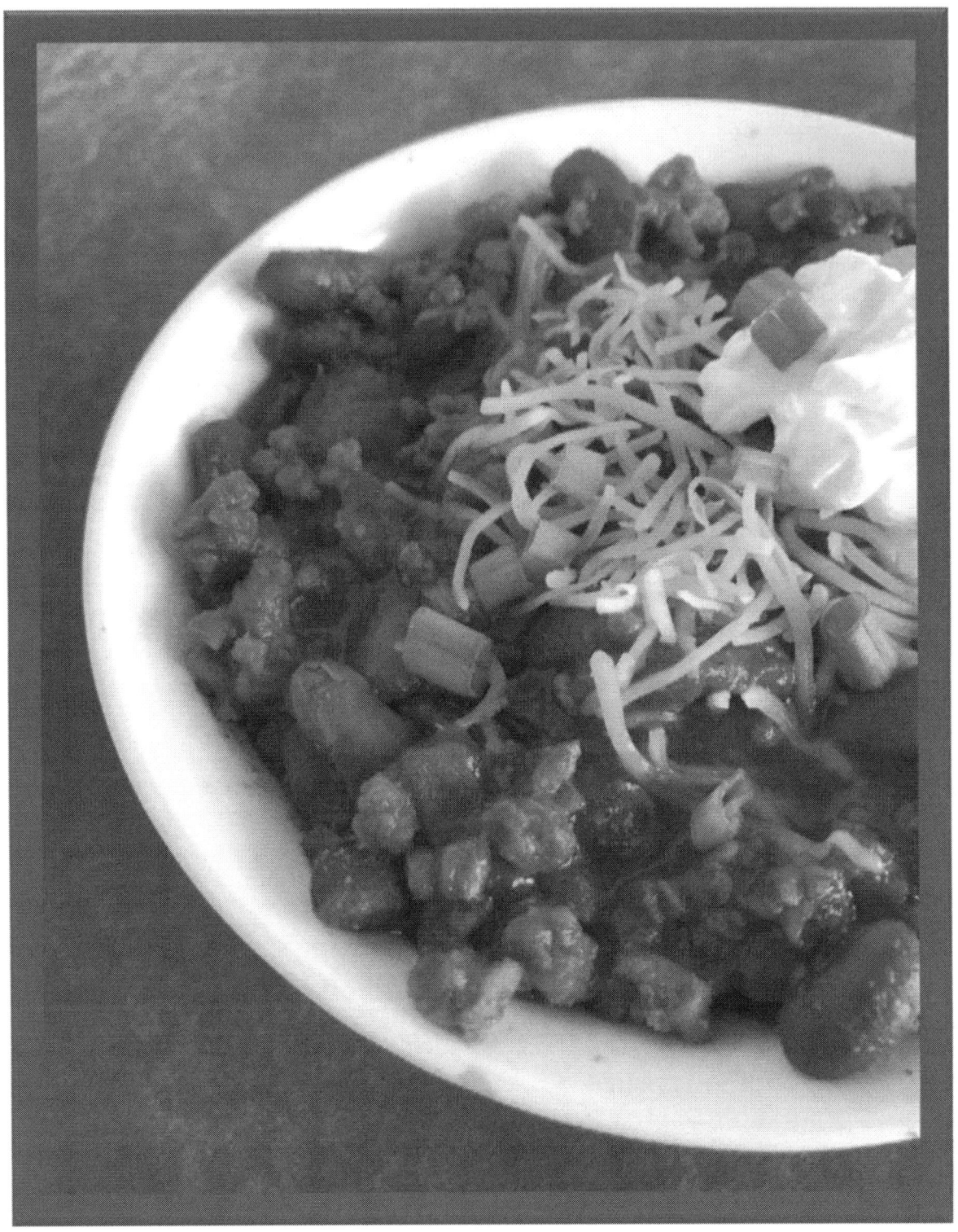

Honey Sesame Chicken

Serves: 4
6 SmartPoints™

Ingredients:
1 pound boneless, skinless chicken breast
2 teaspoons coconut oil
½ teaspoon salt
1 teaspoon coarse ground black pepper
½ teaspoon cayenne powder
1 tablespoon freshly grated ginger
2 tablespoons honey
¼ cup soy sauce
2 teaspoons sesame oil
1 tablespoon sesame seeds, toasted (optional)
Fresh lemongrass for garnish, optional
Cooked rice for serving (optional)

Directions:
1. Using a meat mallet, flatten the chicken until it is approximately ¼ inch thick.
2. Melt the coconut oil in a skillet over medium heat.
3. Season the chicken with salt, black pepper, and cayenne powder. Cook the chicken in the skillet for 4-5 minutes per side, or until it is no longer pink in the center.
4. In a small bowl, combine the fresh ginger, honey, soy sauce, and sesame oil. Mix well and pour the sauce over the chicken.

Delicious Chicken Fried Rice

Serves: 4
4 SmartPoints™
Ingredients:
4 large egg whites
12 ounces boneless, skinless chicken breast, cut in ½ -inch pieces
½ cup carrot, diced
½ cup scallion (green and white parts), chopped
2 garlic cloves, minced
½ cup frozen green peas, thawed
2 cups cooked brown rice, hot
3 tablespoons soy sauce (low-sodium)

Directions:

1. Coat a large, nonstick skillet with cooking spray, and set it over medium-high heat.
2. Add the egg whites and stir frequently as you cook, until they are scrambled, about 3-5 minutes. Place the eggs on a plate and set them aside.
3. Remove the pan from the heat and coat it again with cooking spray and place it over medium-high heat.
4. Add the chicken and carrots and sauté for about 5 minutes or until the chicken is golden brown. Check that the chicken is cooked through before adding the other ingredients.
5. When the chicken is ready, add the chopped scallions, minced garlic, peas, cooked brown rice, the egg whites, and soy sauce. Stir until the ingredients have combined well and continue cooking until all the ingredients are well heated.
6. Serve and enjoy.

Nutritional Information:
Calories 178, Total Fat 2.0 g, Saturated Fat 0.8 g, Total Carbohydrate 21.0 g, Dietary Fiber 38.0 g, Sugars 2.0 g, Protein 18.0 g

Tasty Orange Chicken

Serves: 4

3 SmartPoints™

Ingredients:

2 teaspoons olive oil or cooking spray

¾ cup sweet yellow onion, sliced

1 cup red bell pepper, sliced

1 pound boneless, skinless chicken breast, cubed

½ teaspoon salt

1 teaspoon coarse ground black pepper

1 teaspoon garlic powder

¼ cup low sugar orange marmalade

2 tablespoons soy sauce

Cooked rice for serving (optional)

Directions:

1. Heat the olive oil or cooking spray in a skillet over medium heat.
2. Place the onion and red bell pepper in the skillet and cook for 3-5 minutes, or until the vegetables are just starting to become tender. Remove from the skillet and set aside.
3. Season the chicken with the salt, black pepper and garlic powder. Add the chicken to the skillet and cook, stirring occasionally, for 5-7 minutes.
4. While the chicken is cooking, combine the marmalade and soy sauce. Mix well and then add to the chicken. Toss to coat.
5. Add the vegetables back into the skillet and continue to cook for an additional 5-7 minutes, or until the chicken is cooked through.
6. Remove from the heat and serve warm with cooked rice, if desired.

Nutritional Information:

Calories 173, Total Fat 3.1 g, Saturated Fat 0.8 g, Total Carbohydrate 8.4 g, Dietary Fiber 0.9 g, Sugars 4.6 g, Protein 26.4 g

Chicken and Sweet Potato

Serves: 4
5 SmartPoints™

Ingredients:
2 teaspoons olive oil or cooking spray
4 cups sweet potatoes, peeled and shredded
1 cup sweet yellow onion, diced
1 cup red bell pepper, diced
1 teaspoon salt
1 teaspoon black pepper
1 teaspoon Cajun seasoning mix
2 cups boneless skinless chicken breast, cooked and shredded
2 cups tomatoes, chopped
Fresh scallions, sliced for garnish (optional)

Directions:
1. Heat the olive oil or cooking spray in a large skillet over medium-high heat.
2. In a bowl, combine the sweet potatoes, onion, and red bell pepper. Toss to mix.
3. Add the vegetable mixture to the skillet and cook for 5-7 minutes, stirring frequently.
4. Season the vegetables with salt, black pepper and Cajun seasoning. Using a spatula, press the vegetables firmly into the bottom of the pan. Reduce the heat to medium and let them cook, without disturbing them, for 5-7 minutes, or until a crust begins to form on the bottom of the vegetables.

Spiced Pork with Apples

Serves: 6
5 SmartPoints™
Ingredients:
2 (14 ounce) pork tenderloins
Olive oil cooking spray
2 teaspoon 5-spice powder, divided
2 apples, cored and sliced
1 red onion, sliced
Directions:
1. Preheat the oven to 450°F. Remove any excess fat from the pork.
2. Line the baking pan with foil. Spray the foil lightly with olive oil cooking spray. Sprinkle 1 teaspoon 5-spice powder on the pork tenderloins and then place them on the baking pan. Roast the pork for about 20 to 30 minutes, or until it is ready.
3. Meanwhile, spray a non-stick pan with cooking spray and sauté the sliced onion until tender. Add 1 teaspoon 5-spice powder and mix well. Add the apple slices and sauté again until the mixture becomes soft and the onions are cooked. Cut the pork tenderloins into ½-inch slices and top them with the apple and onion mixture. Serve.

Nutritional Information:
Calories 253, Total Fat 9.3 g, Saturated Fat 3.2 g, Total Carbohydrate 9.2 g, Dietary Fiber 1.7 g, Sugars 4.1 g, Protein 31.9 g

Pork Chops with Salsa

Serves: 4

4 SmartPoints™

Ingredients:

4 ounces boneless pork loin chops (lean), trimmed

Cooking spray

⅓ Cup salsa

2 tablespoons lime juice, freshly squeezed

¼ cup fresh cilantro or parsley, chopped

Directions:

1. Place the chops on a flat surface and press each one of them with the palm of your hand to flatten them slightly.
2. Coat a large, nonstick skillet with cooking spray. Place it over high heat until the oil becomes hot. Add the chops to the skillet and cook each side for 1 minute, or until they are colored medium-brown. Reduce the heat to medium-low.
3. Mix the salsa and the fresh lime juice together and pour the mixture over the chops. Simmer, uncovered for about 8 minutes or until the chops are cooked through.
4. Garnish the chops with chopped cilantro or parsley (if desired). Serve.

Nutritional Information:

Calories 184, Total Fat 8.0 g, Saturated Fat 12.0 g, Total Carbohydrate 2.0 g, Sugars 0.6 g, Protein 25.0 g

Authentic Italian Steak Rolls

Serves: 4
5 SmartPoints™

Ingredients:

1 pound flank steak, thinly sliced in sheets
¼ cup low fat Italian salad dressing
1 cup red bell pepper, sliced
½ pound asparagus spears, trimmed
1 cup onion, sliced
Cooking spray
1 teaspoon salt
1 teaspoon black pepper
Kitchen twine

Directions:

1. Place the steaks in a bowl and cover them with the Italian salad dressing. Toss to coat. Set aside for 15 minutes.
2. Preheat the oven to 350°F and line a baking sheet with aluminum foil.
3. Remove the meat from the marinade and lay the slices out on a flat surface. Season with salt and black pepper as desired.
4. Place the red bell pepper, asparagus and onion pieces on the center of each piece of meat in equal amounts.
5. Roll up each piece of meat around the vegetables and secure with kitchen twine.
6. Heat the cooking spray in a skillet over medium high.
7. Add the steak rolls to the skillet and sear on all sides.
7. Transfer the steak rolls to the baking sheet. Place it in the oven and bake for 15-20 minutes, or until the meat is cooked through and the vegetables are crisp tender.
8. Remove from the oven and let rest 5 minutes before serving.

Nutritional Information:

Calories 211, Total Fat 8.6 g, Saturated Fat 3.7 g, Total Carbohydrate 7.9 g, Dietary Fiber 1.9 g, Sugars 1.8 g, Protein 24.6 g

Tender Beef Soba Bowls

Serves: 4
8 SmartPoints™

Ingredients:

1 pound flank or skirt steak, thinly sliced
Cooking spray
1 teaspoon salt
1 teaspoon black pepper
1 teaspoon ground ginger
4 cups fresh snow peas, washed and trimmed
¼ cup soy sauce
1 cup beef stock
½ pound soba noodles, cooked
Fresh cilantro for garnish (optional)
Lime wedges for garnish (optional)

Directions:

1. Spray a large skillet with vegetable oil and heat over medium.
2. Add the steak slices and season with salt, black pepper, and ground ginger. Cook, stirring occasionally, for 5-7 minutes, or until the meat has reached the desired doneness.
3. Remove the steak from the pan and keep it warm.
4. Add the snow peas to the pan and sauté for 2-3 minutes.
5. Combine the beef stock and soy sauce and add them to the skillet. Cook for 2-3 minutes, or until the liquid comes to a low boil.
6. Add the cooked soba noodles and toss. Cook an additional 1-2 minutes, or until warmed through.
7. Transfer the noodles, broth, and snow peas to a serving bowl and top with slices of steak.
8. Garnish with fresh cilantro and lime wedges before serving, if desired.

Nutritional Information:

Calories 328, Total Fat 8.8 g, Saturated Fat 3.7 g, Total Carbohydrate 31.1 g, Dietary Fiber 2.1 g, Sugars 3.5 g, Protein 32.7 g

Baked Artichoke Chicken

Serves: 4
3 SmartPoints™
Ingredients:
1 pound chicken breast tenders
Cooking spray
1 teaspoon salt
1 teaspoon coarse ground black pepper
1 cup jarred artichoke hearts
1 cup heirloom tomatoes, chopped
3 cloves garlic, crushed and minced
½ cup fresh basil, torn
1 tablespoon olive oil
Directions:
1. Preheat the oven to 375°F and spray an 8x8 or larger baking dish.
2. Place the chicken tenders in an even layer in the baking dish and season with the salt and coarse ground black pepper.
3. Combine the artichoke hearts, tomatoes, garlic, and basil in a bowl. Drizzle in the olive oil and toss to mix.
4. Spread the artichoke mixture over the chicken.
5. Place in the oven and bake for 25-30 minutes, or until the chicken is cooked through.
6. Remove from the oven and let rest at least 5 minutes before serving.

Nutritional Information: *Calories 185, Total Fat 3.2 g, Saturated Fat 0.8 g, Total Carbohydrate 8.9 g, Dietary Fiber 2.0 g, Sugars 1.5 g, Protein 28.4 g*

Herb & Garlic Thai Chicken

Serves: 4
6 SmartPoints™

Ingredients:

1 pound chicken breast tenders
Cooking spray
¼ cup garlic chili sauce
2 tablespoons honey
1 teaspoon salt
1 teaspoon black pepper
2 cups asparagus spears, chopped
1 cup onion, sliced
1 tablespoon olive oil
Cooked rice for serving (optional)

Directions:

1. Preheat the oven to 375°F and spray an 8x8 or larger baking dish with cooking spray.
2. Place the chicken in a single layer in the baking dish and season with the salt and black pepper.
3. In a bowl, combine the garlic chili sauce and honey. Mix well.
4. Pour the sauce mixture over the chicken, using a basting brush to evenly distribute over each piece.
5. Add the asparagus and onion to the baking dish and drizzle with the olive oil.
6. Place the baking dish in the oven and bake for 25-30 minutes, or until the chicken is cooked through.
7. Remove from the oven and let rest for at least 5 minutes before serving.

Nutritional Information:

Calories 242, Total Fat 6.6 g, Saturated Fat 1.3 g, Total Carbohydrate 17.1 g, Dietary Fiber 2.6 g, Sugars 10.6 g, Protein 28.2 g

Pork Tenderloin with Broccoli

Serves 4
7 SmartPoints™

Ingredients

1 pork tenderloin, about 1 pound
Salt and freshly ground black pepper
2 bunches broccoli rabe (about 1 pound), trimmed
Cooking spray
2 tablespoons olive oil, divided
2 tablespoons balsamic vinegar

Directions

1. Preheat oven to the broil setting and set oven rack to the upper-middle position. Line a baking sheet with parchment paper and lightly spray with cooking spray.
2. Trim the pork tenderloin from all visible fat and cut into 8 even slices. Season with salt and pepper on both sides.
3. Place broccoli rabe on the baking sheet. Spray lightly with cooking spray. Place in the oven under the broiler for 6-10 minutes until tender and golden brown. Turn the broccoli rabe over halfway through the cooking, about 4-5 minutes.
4. Warm 1 tablespoon of olive oil in a large heavy bottomed sauté pan like a cast iron over medium-high heat. Fry the pork for 8-10 minutes, turning halfway or until cooked your preferred doneness. Take the pan off the heat and remove the pork to a serving plate. Cover lightly with foil to keep warm.
5. Deglaze the pan with the balsamic vinegar and remaining 1 tablespoon of olive oil. Whisk the bottom of the pan to release the browned bits of flavors into the sauce. Season to taste with salt and pepper.
6. To serve, place 2 slices of the pork tenderloin with a quarter of the broccoli rabe on a serving plate. Pour a quarter of the sauce over the meat and vegetables and serve.

Nutritional Information:

Calories 317, Total Fat 16.1 g, Saturated Fat 3.3 g, Total Carbohydrate 3.8 g, Dietary Fiber 2.8 g, Sugars 0 g, Protein 36.2 g

Supper Easy Pork Piccata

Serves: 4
5 SmartPoints™
Ingredients:
1 pound pork medallions
1 tablespoon olive oil or cooking spray
½ teaspoon salt
1 teaspoon black pepper
2 cloves garlic, crushed and minced
2 tablespoon capers
¼ cup dry vermouth
¼ cup fresh lemon juice
1 tablespoon fresh chives for garnish (optional)
Directions:
1. Heat the olive oil or cooking spray in a skillet over medium heat.
2. Arrange the pork medallions in the skillet and season with salt and black pepper. Cook for 2-3 minutes per side, or until cooked through.
3. Remove the pork medallions from the heat and keep warm until ready to serve.
4. Add the garlic and capers to the skillet. Cook for 1 minute, stirring gently.
5. Add the vermouth and lemon juice. Continue to cook while stirring and scraping the pan for 1-2 minutes.
6. Remove the sauce from the heat and immediately pour it over the pork medallions for serving.
7. Serve garnished with fresh chives, if desired.

Nutritional Information: *Calories 252, Total Fat 9.4 g, Saturated Fat 2.4 g, Total Carbohydrate 0.2 g, Dietary Fiber 0.1 g, Sugars 0.0 g, Protein 33.4 g*

Tender Spiced Pulled Pork

Serves 6
5 SmartPoints™
Ingredients
Rub
1 tablespoon paprika
1-3 teaspoons ancho chili powder according to taste
1 teaspoon salt
1 teaspoon ground cumin
1 teaspoon dry oregano
½ teaspoon black pepper
¼ teaspoon cinnamon
¼ teaspoon dry coriander

Other ingredients
2 pounds pork tenderloin, trimmed
1 onion, diced
4 garlic cloves, minced
1 cup low fat beef broth
1 tablespoon apple cider vinegar

Directions

1. Mix together all the rub ingredients in a small bowl.
2. Rub the spice mix all over the pork
3. Place the garlic, onion, beef broth and apple cider vinegar in the slow cooker. Stir a few times to mix well.
4. Add the pork.
5. Set on LOW and cook for 4-6 hours until the pork is cooked through and shred easily with a fork.

Note: pork can be used to make tacos, sandwiches, and salads.
Nutritional Information:
Calories 190, Total Fat 4.3 g, Saturated Fat 1.2 g, Total Carbohydrate 5.4 g, Dietary Fiber 1.1 g, Sugars 0.9 g, Protein 32.8 g

Hot Curried Pork Chops

Serves: 4
9 SmartPoints™

Ingredients:

1 pound boneless pork chops, approximately ¼ inch thick
Cooking spray
1 teaspoon salt
1 teaspoon black pepper
2 ½ cups carrots, sliced
1 cup unsweetened coconut milk
1 ½ tablespoon curry powder
1 teaspoon lime zest
Cooked rice for serving, optional

Directions:

1. Preheat the oven to 450°F and spray an 8x8 or larger baking dish with cooking spray.
2. Season the pork with salt and black pepper.
3. Place the pork and the sliced carrots in the baking dish, spreading them out into as even a layer as possible.
4. In a bowl, combine the coconut milk, curry powder, and lime zest. Mix well and pour over the pork.
5. Place the baking dish in the oven and bake for 25-30 minutes, or until the pork is cooked through and the carrots are tender.
6. Remove from the oven and let it rest for several minutes before serving.
7. Serve with cooked rice, if desired.

Nutritional Information:

Calories 367, Total Fat 20.1 g, Saturated Fat 7.5 g, Total Carbohydrate 9.9 g, Dietary Fiber 2.2 g, Sugars 3.4 g, Protein 34.9 g

Spicy Pineapple Pork

Serves: 4

8 SmartPoints™

Ingredients:

1 pound cooked pork, shredded

1 tablespoon vegetable oil or cooking spray

3 cups broccoli florets

1 teaspoon salt

1 teaspoon black pepper

2 cups medium heat tomato salsa, fresh or jarred

2 cups fresh pineapple chunks

¼ cup fresh orange juice (or other citrus juice of choice)

Fresh cilantro for serving (optional)

Cooked rice for serving (optional)

Directions:

1. Heat the vegetable oil or cooking spray in a large skillet over medium heat.
2. Add the broccoli and sauté for 5-7 minutes, or until crisp tender.
3. Add the shredded pork to the skillet and season with salt and black pepper.
4. Next, add the salsa, pineapple chunks, and orange juice. Mix well.
5. Increase the heat to medium high until the liquid comes to a low boil.
6. Reduce the heat to low, cover, and simmer for 5-7 minutes, or until heated through.
7. Remove from the heat and serve with cooked rice and cilantro, if desired.

Nutritional Information:

Calories 328, Total Fat 10.3 g, Saturated Fat 2.5 g, Total Carbohydrate 22.7 g, Dietary Fiber 5.0 g, Sugars 9.4 g, Protein 37.4 g

Tender Breaded Veal Cutlets

Serves 4
6 SmartPoints™

Ingredients

1 pound veal cutlets, trimmed
Cooking spray
1/2 cup dry whole-wheat breadcrumbs
1/2 teaspoon paprika
1/2 teaspoon onion powder
1/2 teaspoon salt and black pepper
4 teaspoons canola oil
1 large egg white
4 teaspoons cornstarch

Directions

1. Pound the veal cutlet if needed, so they are ½ inch thick.
2. Preheat oven to 400°F. And line a rimmed baking sheet with parchment paper. Spray lightly with cooking spray.
3. Mix breadcrumbs, and spices in a shallow bowl. Add the oil and mix well.
4. Sprinkle cornstarch over the veal cutlets to evenly coat both sides.
5. Beat the egg white until it becomes frothy. Place in a shallow dish.
6. Add the veal cutlets to the egg white. Massage to coat. Add the cutlets one by one to the breadcrumbs and spices mixt. Try to coat as evenly as possible.
7. Arrange the veal cutlets on the baking sheet. Bake in the preheated oven for 15to 18 minutes, until golden and cooked through.

Nutritional Information:

Calories 219, Total Fat 7 g, Saturated Fat 2.7 g, Total Carbohydrate 11.2 g, Dietary Fiber 1.1 g, Sugars 1.7 g, Protein 24.8 g

Cheesy Fajita Casserole

Serves: 4, 5 SmartPoints™

Ingredients:

½ teaspoon salt

1 teaspoon coarse ground black pepper

1 teaspoon cumin

½ teaspoon cayenne powder

½ teaspoon smoked paprika

Cooking spray

1 pound chicken breast tenders

2 cups yellow and green bell peppers, sliced

1 cup red onion, sliced

1 cup stewed tomatoes, chopped, juice included

¾ cup queso fresco cheese, crumbled

Fresh cilantro for garnish (optional)

Directions:

1. Combine the salt, black pepper, cumin, cayenne powder and smoked paprika. Set aside.
2. Preheat the oven to 375°F and spray an 8x8 or larger baking dish with cooking spray.
3. Arrange the chicken tenders in an even layer in the baking dish and season liberally with at least half of the seasoning mixture.
4. Place the bell peppers and onions over the chicken, followed by the stewed tomatoes.
5. Add any remaining seasoning mixture to the top of the peppers and onions.
6. Sprinkle the queso fresco cheese over the top and place the pan in the oven.
7. Bake uncovered for 25-30 minutes, or until the chicken is cooked through.
8. Remove from the oven and let sit for 5 minutes.
9. Serve warm, garnished with fresh cilantro, if desired.

Nutritional Information:

Calories 233, Total Fat 7.7 g, Saturated Fat 3.8 g, Total Carbohydrate 8.7 g, Dietary Fiber 2.0 g, Sugars 1.5 g, Protein 31.4 g

Tastty Creamy Dijon Chicken

Serves: 4

3 SmartPoints™

Ingredients:

1 pound boneless, skinless chicken breasts

1 tablespoon olive oil or cooking spray

1 teaspoon salt

1 teaspoon white pepper

1 teaspoon fresh thyme

¼ cup Dijon mustard

½ cup low fat milk

2 cloves garlic, crushed and minced

4 cups fresh spinach, torn

Directions:

1. Heat the olive oil in a skillet over medium heat.
2. Using a meat mallet, pound the chicken until it reaches a thickness of approximately ¼ inch.
3. Season the chicken with salt, white pepper and fresh thyme. Add the chicken to the skillet and cook for 3-4 minutes per side.
4. Combine the Dijon mustard, milk, and garlic.
5. Add the Dijon mixture to the skillet and cook for 1-2 minutes.
6. Add the spinach and cook an additional 4-5 minutes, turning the chicken occasionally, until the chicken is cooked through and the spinach is wilted.
7. Remove from heat and serve warm with favorite accompaniment.

Nutritional Information:

Calories 170, Total Fat 3.2 g, Saturated Fat 0.8 g, Total Carbohydrate 2.6 g, Dietary Fiber 0.7 g, Sugars 1.7 g, Protein 27.6 g

Light Chicken Breast Salad

Serves: 3
4 SmartPoints™

Ingredients:

2 pieces boneless chicken breast
2 celery stalks, finely chopped
1 chicken bouillon cube
¼ onion, chopped
3 tablespoons light mayonnaise
2 tablespoons parsley chopped

Directions:

1. Place the chicken breasts, half of the chopped celery, half the onion, and parsley in a medium saucepan. Cover the ingredients with water. Add the chicken bouillon cube, and cover with a lid.
2. Cook on medium heat for about 15 to 20 minutes, or until the chicken has cooked through. Remove the chicken from the heat and let it cool. Reserve the chicken broth.
3. Dice the chicken and place it in a bowl. Add the remaining celery, onions, and the mayonnaise. Add ⅛ cup of the chicken broth you had reserved, and mix well. Add more if the chicken looks dry. Serve on lettuce, as a lettuce wrap, or on bread.

Nutritional Information:

Calories 169, Total Fat 5.3 g, Saturated Fat 2.8 g, Total Carbohydrate 4.1 g, Dietary Fiber 1.0 g, Sugars 1.1 g, Protein 25.4 g

Turkey Mac with Jalapenos

Serves: 8, 8 SmartPoints™

Ingredients:

2 teaspoon chili powder

1 teaspoon garlic powder

1 teaspoon ground coriander

1 teaspoon onion powder

1 teaspoon cumin

¼ teaspoon salt

1 tablespoon olive oil

1 pound ground turkey

3 cups beef broth

1 (10 ounce) can tomatoes with green chilies, diced

2 cups dry whole wheat elbow pasta

½ cup low fat milk

4 ounces cream cheese

1 cup cheddar cheese, shredded

½ cup pickled jalapenos, chopped

Directions:

1. In a small bowl, mix together the chili powder, garlic powder, ground coriander, onion powder, chili powder, cumin, and salt.
2. In a medium saucepan, heat the olive oil on medium-high. Add the turkey and cook until it turns color. Add the spices, mix them in, and allow the mixture to cook for a further 1 or 2 minutes. Stir in the beef broth, diced tomatoes, and dry pasta. Cover the pot and cook for about 8 to 10 minutes.
3. Before the pasta finish cooking, poor the milk in a pot and place it over low heat. When the milk is warm and steamy, mix in the cheese cream until it melts. The shredded cheese can then be added to the milk. Stir until it melts.
4. Empty the cheese sauce into the pasta blend and mix until the pasta is equally covered. Blend in the pickled jalapenos. Give it a taste and add more salt if necessary. Serve hot.

Nutritional Information:

Calories 322, Total Fat 15.0 g, Saturated Fat 4.8 g, Total Carbohydrate 20.3 g, Dietary Fiber 4.0 g, Sugars 11.2 g, Protein 20.0 g

Delicious Grilled Chicken Salad

Serves: 4

6 SmartPoints™

Ingredients:

¼ cup mayonnaise (low-fat)

1 teaspoon curry powder

2 teaspoons water

4 ounces or 1 cup rotisserie chicken, preferably lemon herb flavor, chopped

¾ cup apple, chopped

⅓ Cup celery, diced

3 tablespoons raisins

⅛ Teaspoon salt

Directions:

1. In a medium-sized bowl, combine the mayonnaise, curry powder, and water. Stir with a whisk until well blended.
2. Add the chopped chicken, celery, raisins, chopped apple, and salt. Stir the ingredients so they get combined well. Cover the salad and chill in the fridge. Serve in a lettuce wrap, with bread, or on its own.

Nutritional Information:

Calories 222, Total Fat 5.4 g, Saturated Fat 2.1 g, Total Carbohydrate 26.9 g, Dietary Fiber 2.5 g, Sugars 8.1 g, Protein 23.0 g

Delicious Chicken Salad

Serves: 4
4 SmartPoints™
Ingredients:
2 ½ cups chicken, cooked and chopped
3 stalks celery, chopped
1 cup apple, chopped
¼ cup cranberries, dried
½ cup plain Greek yogurt (nonfat)
2 tablespoons Hellman's mayonnaise, light
2 teaspoons lemon juice
Salt and pepper to taste
Optional:
2 tablespoons fresh parsley, chopped
Directions:

1. In a large bowl, mix the chicken, celery, apple, and dried cranberries. Stir the ingredients and combine them well.
2. In a small bowl, mix the yogurt, mayonnaise, and lemon juice. Add the mixture to the chicken mixture and mix well. Stir in the chopped parsley, if using. Add salt and pepper to taste.
3. Serve on whole grain crackers, rice, pita bread, or make a wrap.

Nutritional Information:
Calories 220 Total Fat 5.0 g, Saturated Fat 1.1 g, Total Carbohydrate 13.0 g, Dietary Fiber 2.0 g, Sugars 7.1 g, Protein 28.0 g

Raspberry Balsamic Chicken

Serves: 3
5 SmartPoints™
Ingredients:
3 pieces boneless skinless chicken breast
¼ cup all-purpose flour
Cooking spray
⅔ Cup chicken broth (low fat)
½ cup raspberry preserve (low sugar)
1 ½ teaspoons cornstarch
1 ½ tablespoons balsamic vinegar
Salt and black pepper to taste
Directions:

1. Cut the boneless and skinless chicken breast into bite-sized pieces. (You may also pound them into thin cutlets to cook through easily.) Season the chicken with salt and black pepper to taste. Dredge the chicken pieces in the flour, and shake off any excess.
2. Heat a non-stick skillet over medium heat and coat it with spray. Cook the chicken for about 15 minutes, turning halfway through so both sides can cook well. Remove the cooked chicken from the skillet.
3. Mix the chicken broth, raspberry preserves, and cornstarch in the skillet over medium heat. Stir in the balsamic vinegar. Add chicken back to the pan. Cook for about 10 minutes, turning halfway through.

Nutritional Information:
Calories 229, Total Fat 4. 6 g, Saturated Fat 0.8 g, Total Carbohydrate 21.8 g, Dietary Fiber 0.7 g, Sugars 15.0 g, Protein 24.5 g

Thank for making it through to the end of *this book*. Let's hope it was informative and able to provide you with all of the tools you need to achieve your weight loss goals.

Michael M

35787668R00081

Made in the USA
Lexington, KY
07 April 2019